Praise for *The Effect of Falun Gong*

"*The Effect of Falun Gong on Health and Wellness* exudes optimism and hope during this global pandemic crisis when many of us, including physicians, are searching for answers. The study from Dr. Trey's findings shows that Falun Gong has much to offer in the overall enhancement of mind-body health and well-being."

—*Dr. Nguyen Nam Binh, Anesthesiologist, Ho Chi Minh City, Vietnam*

"Dr. Trey has put together her experience as a researcher and practitioner of Falun Gong with the scientific description of a researcher and the authentic prescription of a practitioner. In this book, she efficaciously conveys to readers the effectiveness, simplicity, and importance of Falun Gong, not only on health and wellness but also on all dimensions of daily life."

—*Dr. Mahesh Bhatt, Consultant Surgeon, Public Health Researcher, President of VIBHA, and Author of Spiritual Health, Dehradun, Uttarakhand, India*

"Are you searching for a profound change—a way to ease stress, overcome anxiety, and achieve inner joy and equanimity? Dr. Trey's pioneering study shows that people who practice Falun Gong experience better health and wellness than those who do not. Why not give it a try?"

—*Dr. Hiem Van Vo, Associate Director, Board for Hong Ngu Regional General Hospital, Dong Thap, Vietnam*

"As a counselor, Dr. Trey focuses on the realm of clients' perceptions. As a researcher, she makes a sound contribution to the readers' understanding of the effects of Falun Gong by focusing on observing those perceptions. I practice spirituality and meditation and this book has helped me see that practicing Falun Gong can improve one's health in multiple ways."

—*Nora Truscello, International Speaker, Best-Selling Author of* The Science of Intuition, *PA, USA*

"If you are a health professional seeking ways to help concerned patients see that better health, wellness, and improved immunity can be in their own hands, without having to step outside their doors, this book will be extremely helpful. I highly recommend it. Falun Gong is the way to go for better health and wellness."

—*Dr. Nguyen Duc Truong, Obstetrician-Gynecologist, Ho Chi Minh City, Vietnam*

"This is fantastic! Reconnecting with ancient wisdom and revitalizing wellness and health through mind-body practice is the best gift of awareness for everyone. Dr. Trey's book is very much needed in our world today. Embracing a valued meditative practice is imperative to self-worth and healing. Her research findings reveal significant support that Falun Gong can enhance, heal, restore, revive, and provide varied benefits. The modern lifestyle requires essential wellness practices and one of them is the mindfulness practice of Falun Gong. An authentic work and a must-read."

—*Bhavna Khemlani, University Lecturer, Corporate Trainer, Researcher, and Author of Gratitude, Good News & Guidelines Anthology and other novels, Bangkok, Thailand*

"Dr. Trey designed an effective, empirical study that shines light not only on the mental and physical health benefits of practicing Falun Gong, but also on the spiritual benefits. This support of the powerful mind-body-spiritual connection is likely to validate current practitioners, encourage new ones, and stimulate further research. The insight given about integrating meditative practices into counseling makes this a must-read for helping professionals."

—*Amoneeta Beckstein, Ph.D., Counseling Center Director, Psychology Faculty, Webster University Thailand, Cha-am, Bangkok*

"Dr. Trey's research admirably displays her mastery of the tools of her academic trade. She has methodically researched her topic, negotiated the ethics protocol, solicited, and managed a huge amount of data. Above all, her ground-breaking study will help readers to realize that practicing Falun Gong reaps tremendous benefits."

—*Songfa Liu, Ph.D., Earth Scientist, Senior Public Servant, Canberra, Australia*

"As a researcher and Falun Gong practitioner, Dr. Trey presents a comprehensive study on the benefits of Falun Gong practice, combining scientific data and practice, making it easy to read and understand. Her research not only presents a highly persuasive illustration of the beneficial effects of this particular spiritual practice, but it is also another powerful reminder of interconnectedness of mind, body, and spirit, and the importance of a holistic approach to health and wellbeing, while offering evidence of how Falun Gong practice may help to achieve this. This book is a much-needed and well-timed contribution during the current global mind, body, and spirit health crises. I highly recommend it for learning more about the benefits of Falun Gong practice and also as a reminder that the power to heal lies within."

—*Vladimir Mladjenovic, Founder of Tomorrow People Organization, Co-creator of Quarantinestories.world*

The Effect of

FALUN GONG

On Health & Wellness

The Effect of

FALUN GONG

On Health & Wellness

As Perceived by Falun Gong Practitioners

Dr. Margaret Trey

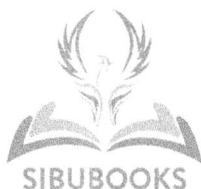

SIBUBOOKS

Sibubooks LLC.
For enquiries, contact us at sibubooks@gmail.com

Editor: Louise Stevanovic
Cover design: Rebeca Covers
Cover image photography: Emma Morley
Interior design and formatting: Louise Stevanovic & Eugene Rijn Saratorio
Ebook formatting: Ankit Todi

Library of Congress Catalogue Number: 2020900096
ISBN: 978-0-9972281-2-0
EBook ISBN: 978-0-9972281-4-4

The Effect of Falun Gong on Health and Wellness as Perceived by Falun Gong Prac-titioners / Dr. Margaret Trey.
1. Energy healing. 2. Integrative counseling. 3. Mind-body therapies. 4. Mindfulness practice. 5. Meditation. 1. Title.

Printed in the United States of America.

To my late mother
who instilled in me the appreciation for
ancient wisdom

To all who see the necessity for
further research on
Falun Gong

UNIVERSITY OF SOUTH AUSTRALIA
Adelaide

A dissertation submitted in partial satisfaction of the
requirements for the degree
Doctor of Counseling

by

Margaret Trey (née Lau)
Doctor of Counseling
University of South Australia, Adelaide, 2010

Dr. John H. Court, 1st Supervisor
Dr. Heather Mattner, 2nd Supervisor

2010

Abstract

The Effect of Falun Gong on Health and Wellness
As Perceived by Falun Gong Practitioners

The promotion of mind-body, health-wellness practices demand ongoing consideration by health professionals as more individuals are seeking alternative therapies and Eastern meditative practices for their health and wellness needs. Falun Gong presents as one such mind-body Eastern meditative spiritual cultivation practice that is gaining worldwide popularity, although knowledge of its effects, potential use in counseling and health-wellness promotion is still lacking. There is a dearth of studies investigating the effects of Falun Gong and limited information about the demographic profile of Falun Gong practitioners around the world. This research provides a demographic profile (excluding mainland China) of Falun Gong practitioners and presents the health-wellness effects of Falun Gong as perceived by Falun Gong practitioners, compared with individuals who do not practice Falun Gong. The research reveals observed similar demographic characteristics between Falun Gong and non–Falun Gong respondents. Both groups mainly comprise married females with tertiary education and professional careers. Falun Gong respondents are just like non–Falun Gong individuals—they are married, and have families and occupations in society, just like other law-abiding citizens, with the exception of their spiritual beliefs and practice, which offers them health-wellness benefits. There are observed differences between the two groups in self-reports of medical history and general health-wellness status. Falun Gong respondents are more likely to report excellent health, no or little use of medication, and less medical and health expenses compared to non–Falun Gong respondents. Falun Gong practice may have public medical and health care implications for the ageing society. The research shows that people who practice Falun Gong have more positive and optimistic perceptions of their health. They report a better health-wellness status than those who do not practice Falun Gong. The findings support Falun Gong as a beneficial mind-body, health-wellness meditative practice.

Contents

Preface

Ten years have passed since I graduated in 2010. In 2012, I had the idea to turn my doctoral dissertation into a book that would be more readable for the public. The search for an academic publisher began and soon culminated in finding a noteworthy Canadian university publisher willing to accept my doctoral-to-book proposition. Another two years fleeted by until finally, in mid-2014 after a change of staff at the publisher, I was told that my book project was "not a good fit" for them.

A turn of events happened in late 2014 when I happened to be in Vancouver, Canada. While there, I attended a book launch for *The Slaughter* by Ethan Gutmann, who rightly advised me to consider self-publishing to get my book out. There is no longer a stigma attached to self-publishing, he said, and these words of encouragement stuck in my mind. Thus, in April 2016, I published *The Mindful Practice of Falun Gong: Meditation for Health, Wellness and Beyond.* My research topic is about Falun Gong, the widespread spiritual practice whose followers have been brutally persecuted in China since 1999. Some publishers are reluctant to risk offending the Chinese regime by publishing such research. To get the book out to the public, I needed to do something myself.

A series of situations led me to consider publishing my dissertation *as is.* People were curious and asked me for my doctoral dissertation. A psychology PhD student from Bulgaria contacted me seeking permission to translate a portion of *The Mindful Practice of Falun Gong* as part of her course requirement. Later, a master's degree student from Germany contacted me about my research for her thesis: *Falun Gong in der Schule - Motive, Umsetzungsformen und Erfahrungen* (translated as Falun Gong in Schools - motives, ways of implementation and experiences). Then came offers to translate *The Mindful Practice of Falun Gong* into several languages, projects that are now in progress for the Chinese and Vietnamese translations.

After nearly a decade since beginning my research, there is still a dearth of studies exploring the effects of Falun Gong. Neither is there development of more academic papers exploring the concept of integrating the spiritual cultivation system into counseling and other helping professions. Hence, I decided to publish the dissertation *as is*, to document a pioneering research endeavor that is not without its limitations. Yet, I believe that my pioneering effort can serve as a beacon for others and be a stepping-stone for future studies on Falun Gong.

The dissertation proper starts in the next section. While the content of the research is kept *as is*, there are pertinent editing changes and URLs updates in the published dissertation. One of the changes involves the arrangement and numbering of the book chapters. The original dissertation comprises only six chapters. Here it is extended to 10 chapters. For instance, the literature review is split into two chapters—one focusing on non–Falun Gong literature and the other on Falun Gong-related literature. Likewise, the original long chapter on findings has been split into four chapters in this book. Chapter 5 covers the findings for Falun Gong respondents, while Chapter 6 presents the findings for non–Falun Gong respondents. Chapter 7 focuses on respondents' written comments and Chapter 8 discusses comparisons between the two groups.

The original dissertation is 256 pages in A4 format. The book format, however, required some materials in the appendices to be removed, making room for three new sections—Updated Resources, a small Index, and About the Author. Apart from updates to out-of-date hyperlinks and DOIs (Digital Object Identifier), the references remain intact. Another change is replacing the word 'thesis' with 'dissertation' throughout the book to be consistent with the U.S. definitions of the two terms.

I wish to thank Professor David Ownby at the University of Montreal for his trailblazing field studies on Falun Gong that inspired me to forge ahead to conduct this research under the auspices of the University of South Australia, as partial fulfillment of my doctorate. Over a decade after completing my doctoral research, Professor Ownby still lends me a helping hand. My sincere appreciation goes to Dr. David Zhang, Amy Duncan, Esther Wang, Nicholas Earle, and the proofreading team that included Christine Ford, Desmond Ford, Beth Jen, Diana Mathias, Orysia McCabe, and Cornelia Ritter for their meticulous review of the manuscript. I remain grateful to poet and editor

Damian Robin, advisor to the Society of Classical Poets, who once again put himself on standby to provide copyediting support. My deepest appreciation goes to the book's editor, Louise Stevanovic, for painstakingly proofreading, copyediting, helping to format the book, and providing overall support in preparing this long overdue book for publishing.

Others who have offered incredible support and helped make a positive difference include Chinese translation book editor Caroline Zhang, Jens Almroth, Michaela Hawkins, my husband Oliver, and my sister Cathy Lau. My heartfelt appreciation goes to Angela Lee, Thanh Nguyen and, in particular, Thao Truong, for their roles in helping me navigate significant turning points in my cultivation journey. I am grateful to these special individuals, and countless others, whose names are not mentioned here, as there are too many to list. Their support and impact have been felt and deeply etched in my heart as I traverse the meandering journey of preparing this dissertation for publication. I thank each one of you from my heart. As we step forward with courage and faith, we know that the invisible Hand is always there to support and guide us. And so, without further ado, I will let the doctoral dissertation *as is* unfold from here.

CHAPTER 1

Introduction

We must close our eyes and invoke a new manner of seeing ... A wakefulness that is the birthright of us all, though few put it to use. (Plotinus, 1975, p.42)

1.1 Chapter overview

Health and wellness are important to everyone. With increasing costs of health care and societal stresses, promoting and maintaining mind-body health and wellness is a challenge that demands ongoing consideration by all health professionals. More individuals are now seeking to sustain their health and wellness through Eastern meditative practices, alternative therapies and options that go beyond traditional medical contexts (Atwood & Maltin, 1991; Delmonte, 1984; Easton, 2005; Krisanaprakornkit, Krisanaprakornkit, Piyavhatkul, & Laopaiboon, 2006; Monk-Turner, 2003; Shapiro Jr., 1980; Singer, 2006; Walsh, 1989; Walsh & Vaughan, 1993). Where new learning can be gained to enhance our knowledge, it is vital to consider the potential and impact of new mind-body practices for improving health-wellness outcomes.

Falun Gong presents itself as one such mind-body Eastern meditative movement and spiritual cultivation practice that is gaining popularity worldwide, although knowledge of its potential for use in counseling and health-wellness promotion is still lacking. Falun Gong is free and considered a bio-psycho-spiritual practice (Kutolowski, 2007). The readers of this dissertation, including counselors, therapists, and other health professionals, are encouraged to consider it with "a new manner of seeing" (Plotinus, 1975, p. 42).

This dissertation presents the findings of the first Australian-based research on the demographic profile of Falun Gong practitioners and their health. It presents a demographic profile of Falun Gong practitioners, an investigation of the health-wellness effects of Falun Gong on practitioners, and their report of perceived health and wellness as compared with non–Falun Gong individuals. The findings of this research highlight the differences between individuals who practice Falun Gong and those who do not in terms of health and wellness outcomes. This dissertation provides an insight into the use of Falun Gong as a self-improvement mind-body technique, an adjunct to counseling, and in health-wellness promotion.

Findings of this research are of significant consequence and relevance to counselors, all health professionals, and members of the public who are receptive to the therapeutic potential of mind-body Eastern meditative movement and spiritual practices. This dissertation offers a resource for all individuals in the helping professions to understand Falun Gong in its cultural, health, and healing contexts, and thus better equip them with the knowledge and understanding to offer appropriate, effective, and sensitive support services to individuals who practice Falun Gong.

1.2 Arrangement of this dissertation

This chapter provides an overview of this dissertation and a synopsis of each chapter. It presents an introduction to Falun Gong, the aims and scope of this research, and definitions of related terms and key concepts. It also introduces the positive link between spirituality/religion and health, which forms the theoretical framework for this research. Chapter 2 presents a comprehensive general literature review on studies and topics related to this research, and provides a critical analysis of this literature. Chapter 3 focuses on the literature review of existing Falun Gong literature, its health and wellness effects, as well as a broader review that includes other Eastern meditative practices, such as tai chi and qigong. Chapter 4 discusses the research design, methodology, and the three phases of the entire research process. It explains the rationale for the choice of research design, the use of self-reporting, the self-designed questionnaires, and the Short Form (SF) 36 Health Survey (Ware Jr., 2008; Ware Jr. & Sherbourne, 1992). Chapters 5 and 6 present the findings of Falun Gong respondents and non-Falun Gong respondents respectively.

There were two components of this research. Part A comprised the demographic profile of Falun Gong respondents compared to non–Falun Gong respondents, and Part B investigated the health-wellness effects of Falun Gong and whether individuals who practice Falun Gong experience better health and wellness than those who do not. Chapter 7 delivers the written comments of the respondents, while Chapter 8 offers a comparison of the findings from two groups of respondents. Chapter 9 presents an analysis and discussion of the findings of this research, attempting to provide insight into possible differences between Falun Gong and non–Falun Gong respondents and the health-wellness effects of Falun Gong. The concluding Chapter 10 gives a synopsis of this dissertation and addresses the limitations and strengths of this research. It offers readers and researchers practical recommendations relating to future studies on Falun Gong, the integration of Falun Gong in counseling practice, and to health-wellness promotion.

1.3 Introduction to Falun Gong

Falun Gong, also known as Falun Dafa, is an ancient Chinese cultivation system for the overall improvement of body, mind, and spirit (Falun Dafa Association, 2009a, 2009b; H. Li, 2001a, 2001b; Parker, 2004; What is Falun Dafa?, 2002). It is a mind-body practice that has ancient roots in traditional Chinese culture. Falun Gong is based on the universal principles of truthfulness, compassion, and forbearance, or *Zhen, Shan, Ren* (H. Li, 2001b, pp. 13-17). (Refer to the Glossary for an explanation of the Chinese terms.) Falun Gong has two distinct components: 1) Cultivating the heart and elevating the mind; and 2) Practicing the physical exercises (H. Li, 2001b). Falun Gong practitioners cultivate their body, mind, and spirit through studying the teachings of Falun Gong regularly, embracing these teachings in their daily lives, and practicing the four standing exercises and one sitting meditation (H. Li, 2001a, 2001b).

Self-cultivation, or simply cultivation, is an Eastern concept for mind, body, and spiritual improvement (Xie & Zhu, 2004). The Chinese term for cultivation is *xiulian; xiu* means "repair," "restore," or "fix," while *lian* means to "improve" or "refine" (Clearwisdom editors, 2006; Life and hope renewed, 2005, p. IV). The cultivation aspect of the mind in Falun Gong practice involves improving *xinxing*, that is, improving one's moral character or one's heart-mind nature by following the three universal principles of truthfulness, compassion, and forbearance in everyday life (Clearwisdom editors, 2006; H. Li, 2001a, 2001b; Life and hope renewed, 2005). Practicing cultivation thus requires cultivating the mind, which is called *xinxing* cultivation (H. Li, 2001b). *Xinxing* includes "virtue (a type of matter), tolerance, enlightenment quality, sacrifice, giving up ordinary people's desires and attachments, being able to suffer hardships" (H. Li, 2001b, p. 28). When *xinxing* is improved, the physical body will undergo transformation (H. Li, 2001b).

The role of karma, the law of cause and effect (H. Li, 2001a, 2001b), is relevant to the health-wellness of Falun Gong practitioners. According to Falun Gong teachings, every illness condition has a corresponding dark or black energy field caused by karma (H. Li, 2001a, 2001b). Besides the improvement of *xinxing*, this karmic energy field has to be eliminated and replaced with a positive energy field or "virtue" before healing can take place (H. Li, 2001b). Falun Gong practitioners will go through body purification, cleansing, elimination, and transformation of the illness karma during cultivation practice, thereby resulting in better health and wellness (H. Li, 2001b).

To cultivate the mind and upgrade *xinxing*, a strong main consciousness is essential, as well as the ability to hold and maintain strong positive and righteous thoughts. Mr. Li Hongzhi, author of the book *Zhuan Falun: The Complete Teachings of Falun Gong*, explained how "the mind must be right" (2001b, p. 245), and how a person can be helped or "be saved and can distinguish good from bad" (2001b, p. 244). Having a right mind in Falun Gong cultivation means being able to always regard oneself as a Falun Gong practitioner and following the three universal principles of truthfulness, compassion, and forbearance (H. Li, 2001b).

Mind-body techniques are referred to as bio-spiritual practices (Kirkland, 1998, 2005; Kutolowski, 2007). Based on the ancient Chinese Taoist system of self-cultivation, a person can transcend the ordinary to become enlightened, or achieve the Tao, through practicing special meditative techniques, and living a moral and virtuous life (Kutolowski, 2007; Xie & Zhu, 2004). Physical exercise is the pathway to the attainment of the Tao. The physical body forms the "basis, the root, the foundation of the cultivation process" (Kutolowski, 2007,

p. 1). Kirkland described this process of transcendental self-transformation as "bio-spiritual self-cultivation" (Kirkland, 1998, p. 3, 2005; Kutolowski, 2007, p. 1). Since the mind corresponds with the psyche, Falun Gong, which is a form of mind-body cultivation, can be considered a Chinese bio-psycho-spiritual self-cultivation system, with its roots in ancient Chinese transcendental practices. The two terms 'bio-spiritual' and 'bio-psycho-spiritual' cultivation will be used synonymously in this dissertation.

The physical aspect of Falun Gong comprises performing five meditative exercises: four simple standing, slowing-moving tai chi-like relaxing exercises, and one sitting meditation (Clearwisdom editors, 2006; Falun Dafa Association, 2009b; Life and hope renewed, 2005; Porter, 2003; What is Falun Dafa?, 2002). Each exercise has specific health-related aims or effects (H. Li, 2001a). Exercise One, known as "Buddha Showing a Thousand Hands" (Fo Zhan Qianshou Fa) (H. Li, 2001a, pp. 141-145), opens up all energy channels, clears congested energy, and stimulates the energy in the body to absorb energy from the universe. The second exercise, "Falun Standing Stance" (Falun Zhuang Fa) (H. Li, 2001a, pp. 145-146), is a tranquil standing meditation comprising four wheel-like holding postures. It awakens inner wisdom and increases strength and energy levels. Exercise Three, known as "Penetrating the Two Cosmic Extremes" (Guantong Liangji Fa) (H. Li, 2001a, pp. 147-152), purifies the body through the blending of energy from the human body and the cosmos, while Exercise Four, "Falun Heavenly Circuit" (Falun Zhoutian Fa) (H. Li, 2001a, pp. 153-155), improves overall circulation and harmonizes anomalous conditions in the body. The fifth exercise, "Strengthening Divine Powers" (Shentong Jiachi Fa), is a sitting meditation that refines the mind and body through *ding* (the optimum state of tranquility), and strengthens divine powers and energy potency (H. Li, 2001a, pp. 155-160).

Mr. Li Hongzhi, the founder of Falun Gong, first introduced Falun Gong as a form of qigong practice to the public in mainland China in the city of Changchun in May 1992, and then to the rest of the world in 1995 (Ownby, 2008a; D. Palmer, 2007; Parker, 2004; Penny, 2001; Porter, 2003). Between 1992 and 1995, Mr. Li Hongzhi conducted 54 public lectures in mainland China (Ownby, 2001; Xie & Zhu, 2004), all of which were organized by the Chinese Communist Party's (CCP) qigong organization called the China Qigong

Scientific Research Society (Parker, 2004; The journey of Falun Dafa, 2002). Within a short period, Falun Gong became one of the most popular qigong practices in mainland China (Falun Dafa Information Center, 2008). Different sources have attributed the initial appeal of Falun Gong to its healing potential and health-wellness effects (Ackerman, 2005; Kutolowski, 2007; Ownby, 2001, 2008a; S. J. Palmer, 2003; Porter, 2003; Pullen, 2000; Wang et al., 1998; Xie & Zhu, 2004; Yang & Nania, 2001; Zhang & Xiao, 1996).

Falun Gong sources stated that a 1998 survey by the CCP established that there were about 70 million Falun Gong practitioners in mainland China (The journey of Falun Dafa, 2002). The CCP later claimed the figure to be about 2 million followers (Ownby, 2001). Penny (2003) commented that the real figures would be impossible to ascertain as practitioners do not have to officially register or join Falun Gong to practice Falun Gong. According to the Falun Gong website, www.falundafa.org, Falun Gong is practiced in over 100 countries and by nearly 100 million people from all walks of life (Falun Dafa Association, 2009a, 2009b)

1.4 Falun Gong: Qigong, spiritual cultivation, or Chinese religious practice

This section discusses the numerous terms used to describe Falun Gong. An explanation for the banning and persecution of Falun Gong in mainland China by the CCP is also presented. Falun Gong has been described with many different terms (Porter, 2003). It has been referred to as a form of qigong (Burgdoff, 2003; Q. Li, Li, Garcia, Johnson, & Feng, 2005; Lio et al., 2003; Lowe, 2003; Ownby, 2008a; D. Palmer, 2007; Parker, 2004; Porter, 2003; Spiegel, 2002), a Buddhist qigong (Penny, 2005), an unofficial traditional Chinese religious practice, or a revival of traditional Chinese spiritual practice (Ownby, 2000, 2003a, 2005, 2008a; Penny, 2003), a new religious movement (Irons, 2003; Ownby, 2003b; Porter, 2005; Wessinger, 2003), a cultural movement (Gale & Gorman-Yao, 2003), or a New Age spiritual movement (Ackerman, 2005). The description of Falun Gong is well encapsulated in the words of the Canadian international human rights lawyer David Matas:

*Falun Gong is authentically Chinese, rooted in ancient Chinese traditions.
It is a blend of ancient Chinese spiritual and exercise traditions. As exercise,
it is a form of qi gong, a set of Chinese exercise practices. ... Th[r]ough his
writings, Li Hongzhi managed to articulate a set of beliefs, which reverberates
with the Chinese people, the Chinese soul (Matas, 2009, p. 2).*

In July 1999, when Falun Gong was banned in mainland China (Matas, 2009; Wessinger, 2003) and the persecution of Falun Gong practitioners first began, Falun Gong was described as a cult in a derogatory sense by the CCP (Bruseker, 2000; Irons, 2003; Porter, 2003; Wessinger, 2003) and by Western critics, such as psychologist Margaret Singer, who spoke at the May 2000 Seattle *Cults and Millennium Conference* (Schechter, 2000, p. 32).

There are complex reasons for the banning and persecution of Falun Gong in mainland China by the CCP. Falun Gong practitioners, Falun Gong sources, and Falun Gong websites, such as www.faluninfo.net and www.clearwisdom. net, other authors, journalists, and researcher scholars have given their insights and reasons for the CCP persecution of Falun Gong (Hsia Chang, 2004; Matas, 2009; Ownby, 2008a; Porter, 2003, 2005; Spiegel, 2002). Porter (2003; 2005) provided six reasons in his master's thesis. Speaking at the International Conference on Religious Freedom in China, held by the European Parliament in Brussels on April 15, 2009, Matas (2009) provided his perspective as to why the CCP persecuted Falun Gong practitioners much worse and much more than members of other spiritual beliefs. One of the key reasons was the CCP's perception of Falun Gong as a threat to national security (A. Jacobs, 2009). This perception was triggered by Falun Gong's capability to mobilize 10,000 to 15,000 practitioners for a silent appeal outside the entrance of Zhongnanhai, the CCP's head office in Beijing, on April 25, 1999, to seek redress and recognition of their rights to practice Falun Gong (A. Jacobs, 2009; Matas, 2009; Ownby, 2008b; Porter, 2005). Another reason was the large numbers—Falun Gong's overwhelming popularity and "diverse demographics" (Porter, 2005, p. 63) that included students, professionals, retirees, and high-ranking CCP party members, with the latter perceived as a threat to the then new leader, Jiang Zemin. Falun Gong was estimated to have about 70 million followers and "a group of that size no matter what its beliefs attracts the attention of a repressive government" (Matas, 2009, p. 2). Other reasons included Mr. Li Hongzhi living in the United States and away from the CCP's control; change of leadership from Deng Xiaoping to Jiang; Jiang's personal jealousy and insecurity; rivalry and contention with other qigong masters and Buddhists in mainland China; and Falun Gong's lack of organizational structure and amorphous nature, rendering it impossible for the CCP to control (Matas, 2009; Porter, 2003).

There is no general consensus on the classification of Falun Gong, leaving writers, scholars, academics, and many journalists baffled over how to describe it (Madsen, 2000; Ownby, 2008a; Porter, 2003). David Ownby (2008a), history professor at the University of Montreal, Canada, discussed the difficulty of explaining Falun Gong and the problem with Falun Gong literature prior to the time of the CCP's persecution of Falun Gong. Like Porter (2003), Ownby (2008a) also provided a comprehensive review and resource of Falun Gong literature. Ownby (2000; 2003a; 2008a) presented a convincing argument in describing Falun Gong in its broader context as a modern Chinese popular religion and a revival of Chinese spiritual traditions. Penny (2003; 2005) and other writers (Bruseker, 2000; Wessinger, 2003) also placed Falun Gong within the same context of Chinese religious traditions in their writings. Richard Madsen (2000), Professor of Sociology at the University of California, San Diego, stated that Falun Gong, which translates as "Dharma wheel practice," is "indeed primarily a practice, something one does rather than something one believes" (p. 243), yet it is considered more akin to a religion because of its reference to Taoism and Buddha Law teachings. Madsen (2000) explained the concept of energy, or *qi,* in the Chinese language. The aim of practicing cultivation is to activate and open up energy channels in the body to promote self-healing, health, and wellness (H. Li, 2001a; Madsen, 2000).

However, Mr. Li Hongzhi makes a clear distinction between *qi* and *gong,* stating that the latter is a "high-energy substance that manifests in the form of light, and its particles are fine and its density is high" (H. Li, 2001a, p. 5). In other words, only *gong* and the cultivation of *gong* will promote genuine healing, and mind-body spiritual transformation (H. Li, 2001a, 2001b). More importantly, Madsen (2000) referred to the ancient Chinese bio-psycho-spiritual philosophy of the interconnectedness of matter and spirit, mind and body, a concept that Mr. Li Hongzhi reiterated as "matter and mind are one thing" (2001b, p. 28). To promote this mind-body, health-wellness concept, physical exercises must be coupled with spiritual or moral cultivation (Kirkland, 1998, 2005; Kutolowski, 2007; Madsen, 2000; Ownby, 2008b; Porter, 2005), a unique feature of Falun Gong. As Ownby (2003b) puts it, Falun Gong is "profoundly moral" (p. 307).

The English translations of the two main texts of Falun Gong are *Falun Gong: Principles and exercises for perfect health and enlightenment* (H. Li, 2001a) and *Zhuan Falun: The Complete Teachings of Falun Gong* (H. Li, 2001b). Falun Gong is frequently referred to in *Lunyu,* or the preface, and throughout the texts as the "Buddha Fa" (H. Li, 2001a, 2001b, pp. 13-15), which is translated as Buddha law, Buddha way, or principles. It is referred to as "an advanced cultivation method of the Buddha School" (H. Li, 2001a, p. 1) and "one of the eighty-four thousand cultivation ways in the Buddha School" (H. Li, 2001b, p. 38). Hence, Falun Gong is richly intertwined with Taoist and Buddhist teachings (H. Li, 2001a, 2001b).

Falun Gong practitioners, and also the CCP, did not describe Falun Gong as a religion (Ownby, 2008a) because the word "religion" does not exist in the Chinese language (Ownby, 2008a; Porter, 2003). Ownby (2008a) offered a succinct explanation in his book *Falun Gong and the future of China* that spiritual cultivation and qigong practices, such as Falun Gong, are not defined as a religion, even though the teachings of Falun Gong embody some religious characteristics. Porter (2003) also provided an insightful argument to the question, "Is Falun Gong a religion?" (pp. 35-40), with an illuminating literature review on the classification of Falun Gong in his master's thesis, published in a book entitled *Falun Gong in the United States: An ethnographic study.* His thesis focused on defining Falun Gong through ethnography, using a variety of research methods to study a Falun Gong community in a specific region in the United States and also via the Internet (Porter, 2003).

Penny (2005) recommended that it is "best to use the Falun Gong terminology to avoid confusion" (p. 38) when describing Falun Gong. To maintain reality and authenticity in the portrayal of Falun Gong through the perceptions of Falun Gong practitioners, this dissertation has consistently adopted Penny's (2005) recommendation, while respectfully presenting the views of other writers and researchers as well. Researchers, such as Burgdoff (2003), S. J. Palmer

(2003), Ownby (2003b; 2008a), and Porter (2003), in conducting fieldwork for their respective Falun Gong studies, took a specific and somewhat similar approach. They immersed themselves in Falun Gong by reading its teachings, attending Falun Gong experience-sharing conferences, building rapport with practitioners, visiting practice sites, joining in the Falun Gong exercise classes, or even marching alongside Falun Gong practitioners (Burgdoff, 2003; Ownby, 2008a; S. J. Palmer, 2003; Porter, 2003).

There is thus a common understanding among writers and researchers that Falun Gong is a form of qigong, a type of spiritual meditation practice, a quasi-religious practice, or a new Chinese religious movement (Ackerman, 2005; Bruseker, 2000; Hu, 2003; Irons, 2003; Madsen, 2000; Ownby, 2000, 2003a, 2005, 2008a; D. Palmer, 2007; S. J. Palmer, 2003; Porter, 2003, 2005; Spiegel, 2002; Wessinger, 2003).

Human Rights Watch author Mickey Spiegel (2002) aptly described Falun Gong as a combination of many qualities:

> A form of qigong, an ancient Chinese deep-breathing exercise system sometimes combined with meditation that enthusiasts claim promotes physical, mental, and spiritual well-being by enhancing the flow of vital energy through a person's body. It also includes elements of popular Buddhism and Daoism (Spiegel, 2002, p. 8).

It is important to stress that Falun Gong, sometimes called "Chinese yoga" (Parker, 2004, p. 40), was first introduced to the public as a form of qigong (Ownby, 2008a; D. Palmer, 2007; Porter, 2003), not as a religion. Mr. Li Hongzhi (2001a; 2001b) stated that Falun Gong is an advanced form of practice, a form of qigong that is "genuinely guiding people to high levels" (2001b, p. 1). Taiwan and U.S. researchers also described Falun Gong as a form of qigong (Q. Li et al., 2005; Lio et al., 2003). To gain a deeper insight into Falun Gong, it is necessary to understand Falun Gong within the context of qigong and the rise and evolution of qigong in mainland China (Ownby, 2000, 2008a; D. Palmer, 2007).

The recognition of Falun Gong as a new Chinese religious movement, a form of qigong, a meditation and cultivation practice for mind-body and spiritual self-improvement is consistent with the aims and scope of this research. Therefore, the link between spirituality/religion and health forms the overarching theoretical framework for this dissertation, and this is discussed further in this chapter.

1.5 Aims and scope of this research

The primary aim of this research is to investigate the health-wellness effects of Falun Gong, as perceived by Falun Gong practitioners, and whether individuals who practice Falun Gong experience better health and wellness than those who do not. "Health" and "wellness" used in this research are as defined by the World Health Organization (WHO) (B. J. Smith, Tang, & Nutbeam, 2006; World Health Organization, 2003). (Refer to Section 1.7 for the definitions of these two terms.)

The secondary aims of this research are:
- To obtain an international demographic profile of Falun Gong practitioners; and
- To ascertain any observed differences or similarities between Falun Gong and non–Falun Gong respondents regarding their demographic profile and health-wellness statuses.

This research is not an investigation of Falun Gong, nor is it about how Falun Gong should be classified. Similarly, this research is not an ethnographic, historical, or socio-political study of Falun Gong. Authors and researchers like Ownby (2003b; 2008a), Porter (2003), and others (Bruseker, 2000; Burgdoff, 2003; Lowe, 2003; S. J. Palmer, 2003) have achieved well in these areas. This research does not investigate the CCP's persecution and torture of Falun Gong practitioners in mainland China (World Organization to Investigate the Persecution of Falun Gong, 2004), human rights issues (Spiegel, 2002), or the reports of organ harvesting of Falun Gong practitioners in China's forced labor camps (Matas & Kilgour, 2006, 2007).

This first Australian-based research is a pioneering study in investigating the health-wellness effects of Falun Gong. Although there have been scholarly studies on Falun Gong (Bruseker, 2000; Burgdoff, 2003; Lowe, 2003; Ownby,

2003b, 2008a, 2008b; S. J. Palmer, 2003; Porter, 2003, 2005), there is a dearth of studies investigating the health-wellness effects of Falun Gong. A Taiwanese study (Lio et al., 2003) used the Short Form (SF-36) Health Survey to examine the health-wellness effect of Falun Gong practice. Besides this study, there were two studies in the United States: one by a group of Falun Gong practitioners (Authors Unknown, 1999; North America Dafa disciples, 2003); and the second by a team of medical doctors (Q. Li et al., 2005). Lau (2001) examined counselors' burnout using Falun Gong as the alternative coping strategy, for a partial fulfillment of the University of South Australia Master's Degree in Social Science (Counselling). This single-case study, completed in Boston (U.S.), showed how Falun Gong, a spiritual cultivation practice, buffered the negative effects of burnout (Lau, 2001).

The research for this dissertation expands on and contributes to the existing few studies on the health-wellness effects of Falun Gong. It is the first such doctoral study that involves a comparison group and investigates whether individuals who practice Falun Gong experience better health and wellness than those who do not. Other studies on Falun Gong (Bruseker, 2000; Lowe, 2003; Ownby, 2003b, 2008a; S. J. Palmer, 2003; Porter, 2003, 2005) did not have a specific health and wellness focus.

1.6 Theoretical framework for this research

This research is based on the premise that spirituality/religion plays a vital role in the health-wellness of individuals who are involved in spiritual or religious practices. It recognizes that spiritual/religious beliefs and practices can have a significant and lasting impact on health and wellness. Falun Gong fits as a bio-psycho-spiritual meditation practice with religious elements from Buddhist and Taoist teachings (Kutolowski, 2007), and it promotes physical, mental, and spiritual health and wellness (Clearwisdom editors, 2006; Gale & Gorman-Yao, 2003; Life and hope renewed, 2005; McCoy & Zhang, n.d.; Spiegel, 2002). Being healthy and well implies having a healthy body, mind, and spirit based on the WHO definitions for health and wellness (B. J. Smith et al., 2006; World Health Organization, 2003, 2007).

There is an increasing body of scientific studies exploring the link between spirituality/religion and health (Koenig, 2004a, 2007; Williams & Sternthal, 2007). D'Souza (2007), director of Clinical Trials and Bipolar Program at the University of Melbourne, and a pioneer in the integration of spirituality in psychiatry and mental health, discussed the beneficial role of spirituality/religion and its use in medical practice. Koenig (1999), co-director of the Center for Spirituality, Theology and Health and Professor of Psychiatry at the Duke University Medical Center, indicated in his book *The healing power of faith: Science explores medicine's last great frontier* that spiritual/religious individuals tend to live longer, have healthier lifestyles, and possess better coping skills, stronger immune systems, and protection from serious cardiovascular illness.

Numerous scientific studies demonstrated the positive link between spirituality/religion and health (Coruh, Ayele, Pugh, & Mulligan, 2005; Haynes, Hilbers, Kivikko, & Ratnavuyha, 2007; Hilbers, Haynes, Kivikko, & Ratnavuyha, 2007; Koenig, 1999, 2004a, 2004b, 2007; Koenig & Cohen, 2002; Koenig, E., & Larson, 2001; Maselko & Kubzansky, 2006; Peach, 2003; Williams & Sternthal, 2007). In fact, the self-healing benefits and the health-wellness promoting potential of Falun Gong was one of the explanations for the rapid growth and widespread popularity of Falun Gong (Life and hope renewed, 2005; S. J. Palmer, 2003). Falun Gong was granted the "Star Qigong School" award as the "most outstanding qigong practice" (H. Li, 2001b, p. 293) in the Beijing state-run Oriental Health Expo in 1992 (Ownby, 2003a).

Mr. Li Hongzhi has described Falun Gong as a high-level qigong and spiritual cultivation practice (H. Li, 2001b), that involves both mind and body cultivation, with an emphasis on cultivating and improving one's *xinxing* (heart-mind nature or moral character) through adhering to the Falun Gong principles of truthfulness, compassion, and forbearance (H. Li, 2001a, 2001b). Various academics, researchers, and scholars describe Falun Gong as a new Chinese religious movement (Bruseker, 2000; Irons, 2003; Ownby, 2000, 2003a, 2005, 2008a; Porter, 2003, 2005; Wessinger, 2003) or a Buddhist qigong practice (Penny, 2005). Nova Religio Falun Gong symposium dedicated eight articles to Falun Gong in its Journal of Alternative and Emergent Religions, recognizing Falun Gong as "a new religious movement that is being persecuted in the People's Republic of China" (Wessinger, 2003, p. 215).

This research is not measuring spirituality/religion or the causal effects of Falun Gong on health. It is a new study that serves to present another perspective on the link between spirituality/religion and health in its focus on Falun Gong (perceived by many as a new religion/spiritual practice) and its possible health-wellness effects.

1.7 Definitions of terms and key concepts

The main terms and key concepts that are mentioned in this dissertation are defined and explained in this section, and the Chinese terms are explained in the Glossary. They include health, wellness, meditation, complementary and alternative medicine (CAM), Mind-Body Medicine (MBM), psychoneuro-immunology (PNI), and the definitions of, and distinction between, the terms spirituality and religion.

The revised edition of the Oxford Dictionary (2005) defines health as "the state of being free of illness or injury" and "a person's mental or physical condition" (p. 801). These definitions correspond with the World Health Organization's (WHO) definition. Since 1948, the WHO defined health as "a state of complete physical, mental and social well-being and not merely the absence of disease or infirmity" (Hattie, Myers, & Sweeney, 2004, p. 354; Witmer & Sweeney, 1992, p. 140; World Health Organization, 2003, 2007). Likewise, mental health is not just the absence or non-occurrence of mental illnesses. The WHO has defined mental health as a "state of well-being in which the individual realizes his or her own abilities, can cope with the normal stresses of life, can work productively and fruitfully, and is able to make a contribution to his or her community" (World Health Organization, 2007). Wellness was later added to the *WHO Health Promotion Glossary* (B. J. Smith et al., 2006) of new terms, which defines wellness as the:

> *Optimal state of health of individuals and groups. There are two focal concerns: the realization of the fullest potential of an individual physically, psychologically, socially, spiritually and economically, and the fulfilment of one's role expectations in the family community, place of worship, workplace and other settings (cited in B. J. Smith et al., 2006, p. 5).*

Different wellness pioneers and experts, such as Halbert Dunn, M.D. (1961) (cited in Swinford, 1989; cited in Westphal, 1989), William Hettler, M.D. (1984) (Hattie et al., 2004; Jane E. Myers & Sweeney, 2005a), Donald Ardell (1986; Westphal, 1989), and John Travis, M.D. (1988), perceived wellness as a dynamic and developing process. By the mid-1980s, wellness became an accepted term (Ardell, 1986), and counselors recognized it as playing a vital role in health-wellness counseling (Hattie et al., 2004). Wellness is defined from the counseling perspective as a:

> *Way of life oriented toward optimal health and well-being, in which body, mind, and spirit are integrated by the individuals to live life more fully within the human and natural community. Ideally, it is the optimum state of health and well-being that each individual is capable of achieving (Jane E. Myers & Sweeney, 2005b, p. 9; Jane E Myers, Sweeney, & Witmer, 2000, p. 252).*

These definitions of health and wellness embody a holistic approach (Hattie et al., 2004; Witmer & Sweeney, 1992), and recognize the intertwined relationship of health and wellness between and within individuals. The terms health and wellness or health-wellness will be used in this dissertation to embody the holistic meanings of the definitions.

Maintenance is defined as the "process of preserving a condition or situation or the state of being preserved" (Oxford Dictionary, 2005, p. 1059). To maintain means to "cause or enable (a condition or situation) to continue, or to keep (something) at the same level or rate" (Oxford Dictionary, 2005, p. 1059). Wellness maintenance can therefore be interpreted as continuing or preserving a way of life that promotes health-wellness outcomes.

Definitions of meditation have many aspects, which include the relaxation response, concentration, focusing the mind on nothing, or on one thought, or an object, or emptying one's thoughts, a changed state of consciousness, and maintaining a state of self-awareness (Perez-De-Albeniz & Holmes, 2000). The word 'meditate' is defined as to "focus one's mind for a period of time, in silence or with the aid of chanting, for religious or spiritual purposes or as a method of relaxation" (Oxford Dictionary, 2005, p. 1091). Meditation thus refers to "the action or practice of meditating" (Oxford Dictionary, 2005, p. 1092).

Two types of meditation have been identified: fixed object or concentrative meditation (CM), and Vipassana meditation, more widely known as insight or mindfulness meditation (MM) (Bogart, 1991; Chambers, Gullone, & Allen, 2009; Goleman, 1976; Krisanaprakornkit et al., 2006; Marlatt & Kristeller, 1999; Naranjo & Ornstein, 1971; Pelletier, 1978; Shapiro Jr., 1980; Walsh & Vaughan, 1993). The difference between the two types of meditation is described here:

> *MM is associated with open monitoring of the entirety of one's experience, and CM is associated with focused attention on a single object, such as a repeated word, or the sensations of breathing, open monitoring may initially involve focused attention (Chambers et al., 2009, p. 561).*

In a comprehensive review of meditation based on 75 articles from 1989 to July 1999, Perez-De-Albeniz and Holmes (2000) summarized the definitions of meditation across different perspectives, ranging from the Webster's dictionary to functional, philosophical, and psycho-physiological descriptions. Pelletier (1978) defined meditation as "an experiential exercise involving an individual's actual attention, not belief system or other cognitive processes" (p. 192), comprising either a "focusing of attention on an object" (p. 192), repeating sacred words such as mantras, or the "opening up of attention" (p. 193). Ornstein (1971), in his chapter discussion on *The Esoteric and Modern Psychologies of Awareness* (pp. 170-212), maintained that meditation can be regarded as "an attempt to turn off conceptual activity temporarily, to shut off all input processing for a period of time, to get away for a while from the external environment" (p. 193). He observed that the goal of Indian, Zen and Sufi meditation was to bring about:

> *An awareness that allows every stimulus to enter into consciousness devoid of our normal selection process, devoid of normal tuning and normal input selection, model building, and the normal category systems (Naranjo & Ornstein, 1971, p. 194).*

Three key words, "awareness-centeredness-emptiness" (Naranjo & Ornstein, 1971, p. 23), can be used to describe the meditation state or the "condition of feelinglessness" (Naranjo & Ornstein, 1971, p. 23). Mr. Li Hongzhi stated that in the Falun Gong sitting meditation, the main consciousness (the conscious mind) must be fully aware and present in the here and now:

> *Your Main Consciousness must be conscious because this practice cultivates your own self. You should make progress with a conscious mind. ... We require of everyone that no matter how deeply you meditate, you must know that you are practicing here. You're absolutely forbidden to be in a state of trance wherein you know nothing. Then, what specific state will occur? When you sit there, you should feel wonderful and very comfortable as though you are sitting inside an egg shell; you will be aware of yourself practicing the exercise, but you feel your whole body cannot move. This is what must occur in our practice (H. Li, 2001b, p. 339).*

Mr. Li Hongzhi explained the state of *ding* during the meditation practice as the optimal state:

> *There is another state in which as one sits for a while, one finds that the legs are gone, and cannot think where the legs went; the body is also gone; the arms are also gone; the hands are also gone—only the head is left. As one keeps practicing, one finds that the head is gone as well, leaving only one's own mind, a little thought that one is practicing here. ... When one practices in this state, the body is being fully transformed, and it is the optimum state. We thus require you to achieve this state of tranquility (H. Li, 2001b, p. 339).*

Every meditation discipline has a different definition of its practice. Assistant Professor and researcher on the psychology of happiness at the University of Toronto, Adam Anderson, described mindfulness meditation as a fitness workout for the human brain: "It's like training any other muscle in your body. You're developing your brain to cope better with the world" (cited in Easton, 2005, p. 22). Meditation is a form of mental fitness exercise increasingly used by researchers, counselors, and other health professionals (Easton, 2005; Lazar et al., 2005).

Meditation, as described in this dissertation, includes a range of Eastern "meditative movement" (C. E. Rogers, Larkey, & Keller, 2009, p. 246) practices and Eastern spiritual cultivation practices. Meditative movement practices refer to mind-body therapies that combine physical movement or postures with breathing, relaxation, and meditation techniques, such as yoga, tai chi, and qigong (C. E. Rogers et al., 2009). Falun Gong can also be classified as one of them. The terms meditation, meditative practices, Eastern spiritual cultivation practices, Eastern mind-body practices, and meditative movement practices will be used interchangeably and synonymously throughout this dissertation. These meditative movement practices are often considered as self-improvement, self-care techniques (G. D. Jacobs, 2001), self-regulation strategies (Shapiro Jr., 1980), or as Mind-Body Medicine (MBM) by the National Center of Complementary and Alternative Medicine (NCCAM) in the United States under its complementary and alternative medicine (CAM) listings (NCCAM, 2008). Meditation is one of the three most widely used CAM therapies (Mao, Farrar, Xie, Bowman, & Armstrong, 2007).

CAM therapies refer to a wide variety of modalities, techniques and approaches. Bishop and Lewith (2008) provided a comprehensive review of CAM use and reported that the most widely used description was the definition by NCCAM. The NCCAM (2008) website defines CAM as "a group of diverse medical and health care systems, practices, and products that are not generally considered part of conventional medicine." Some researchers described CAM as "interventions neither taught widely in medical schools nor generally available in U.S. hospitals" (Eisenberg et al., 1998, p. 1569; Kessler et al., 2001, p. 262). Others (Mamtani & Cimino, 2002; Zollman & Vickers, 1999) preferred the Cochrane Collaboration definition:

> CAM is a broad domain of healing resources that encompasses all health systems, modalities, and practices and their accompanying theories and beliefs, other than those intrinsic to the politically dominant health system of a particular society or culture in a given historical period. CAM includes all such practices and ideas self-defined by their users as preventing or treating illness or promoting health and wellbeing. Boundaries within CAM and between the CAM domain and that of the dominant system are not always sharp or fixed (Mamtani & Cimino, 2002, p. 369; Zollman & Vickers, 1999, p. 693).

NCCAM offers four main categories of CAM therapies, of which Mind-Body Medicine (MBM) is one. (NCCAM, 2008). Meditation is described as a type of mind-body therapy, or technique, or MBM (Goleman & Gurin, 1993; Pelletier, 2002; Shealy, Norris, & Fahrion, 2002; Peter M Wolsko, Eisenberg, Davis, & Phillips, 2004), or a mind-body intervention (Pelletier, 2002; Sierpina, Levine, Astin, & Tan, 2007). These terms will be used interchangeably in this dissertation to mean the same thing.

Mind-Body Medicine (MBM) is defined on the NCCAM website as:

> *A variety of techniques designed to enhance the mind's capacity to affect bodily function and symptoms. Some techniques that were considered CAM in the past have become mainstream (for example, patient support groups and cognitive-behavioral therapy). Other mind-body techniques are still considered CAM, including meditation, prayer, mental healing, and therapies that use creative outlets such as art, music, or dance (NCCAM, 2008).*

MBM was described as "the new medicine" and a "bio-psycho-social/spiritual" (Johnson & Kushner, 2001, p. 257) approach to illness, health and wellness. Goleman and Gurin (1993) classified MBM as a range of modalities, including meditation and relaxation techniques that utilize the human mind in promoting better physical and emotional health and wellness. They proposed that MBM should exist alongside conventional and mainstream health care system because of their lower costs, lower physical and emotional risks, and higher potential benefits (Goleman & Gurin, 1993).

Jacobs (2001) gave three distinctions between MBM and CAM therapies. The first distinction is that MBM considers that the mind plays a vital part in health and wellness maintenance, and rejects the Cartesian theory of mind and body as separate entities (G. D. Jacobs, 2001). Secondly, while less research has been conducted on CAM, there is a mounting body of evidence on MBM in peer-reviewed journals (G. D. Jacobs, 2001). Thirdly, Jacobs (2001) identified the self-care aspect of MBM and how these therapies could be integrated as a self-help technique with conventional medical treatment. Cardiologist Dr. Herbert Benson, one of the pioneers of MBM, developed the self-care concept, describing it as the "three-legged stool" intervention model

(Faneuli, 1997, p. 2; G. D. Jacobs, 2001, pp. S-84). Each of the three legs of the stool represents an intervention strategy: intervention with the use of drugs; intervention with surgery/medical treatment; and intervention with self-help meditation techniques respectively (G. D. Jacobs, 2001). Thus meditation is included as one of the three strategies for self-care, alongside conventional medical interventions in Benson's model of self health care.

In discussing MBM, it is essential to mention the new scientific discipline of psychoneuroimmunology (PNI) (G. D. Jacobs, 2001). PNI was first introduced by Ader (1980) during his presidential address at the American Psychosomatic Society. PNI refers to the study of the relationship between the mind (psyche), nervous system (neuro), immune system, and health (Johnson & Kushner, 2001; Koenig & Cohen, 2002).

Since the link between spirituality/religion and health forms the theoretical framework of this Falun Gong research, it is necessary to define and distinguish the terms "spirituality" and "religion." Koenig, McCullough and Larson (2001) provided a clear distinction between the two terms.

Religion is described as:

> *An organized system of beliefs, practices, rituals, and symbols designed (a)*
> *to facilitate closeness to the sacred or transcendent (God, higher power, or*
> *ultimate truth/reality) and (b) to foster an understanding of one's relationship*
> *and responsibility to others in living together in a community (Koenig et*
> *al., 2001, p. 18; Moreira-Almeida & Koenig, 2006, p. 844).*

Spirituality is defined as:

> *The personal quest for understanding answers to ultimate questions about*
> *life, about meaning and about relationship to the sacred and transcendent,*
> *which may (or may not) lead to or arise from the development of religious*
> *rituals and the formations of community (Koenig et al., 2001, p. 18).*

Most researchers distinguish between the two terms (Coruh et al., 2005; Haynes et al., 2007; Hilbers et al., 2007; Koenig, 2004a, 2004b; Moreira-Almeida & Koenig, 2006, p. 844; Williams & Sternthal, 2007). Religion is described as institutionalized or organized beliefs, involving formal practices, rituals and doctrines (Haynes et al., 2007; Hilbers et al., 2007; Koenig, 2004b; Moreira-Almeida & Koenig, 2006; Williams & Sternthal, 2007), whereas spirituality carries a broader connotation, having different meanings for different individuals (Haynes et al., 2007; Hilbers et al., 2007; Koenig, 2004a, 2004b; Moreira-Almeida & Koenig, 2006; Williams & Sternthal, 2007). Spirituality is identified as "more fluid, eclectic and individual" than religion (Haynes et al., 2007, p. 2; Hilbers et al., 2007, p. 1).

Many authors and researchers either chose to use the two terms interchangeably (Koenig, 2004b; Rippentrop, Altmaier, Chen, Found, & Keffala, 2005; Weaver, Flannelly, Garbarino, Figley, & Flannelly, 2003), or to not differentiate between them (Williams & Sternthal, 2007). A person can be both spiritual and religious, or spiritual but not religious, or religious and not spiritual (Hilbers et al., 2007). Koenig (2004a) noted that about 90% of patients/clients often described themselves as both spiritual and religious. In interactions with patients/clients, the term "spirituality" is more acceptable, convenient and inclusive, because it does not distinguish between, nor segregate people (Hilbers et al., 2007; Koenig, 2004a, 2004b). Researchers have noted that more studies focused on religious beliefs, practices and assessments of religiosity, rather than on spirituality (Koenig, 2004a, 2004b; Williams & Sternthal, 2007; Yeager et al., 2006). The terms "spirituality" and "religion" will be used interchangeably and synonymously, and referred to as spirituality/religion throughout this dissertation.

1.8 Summary

This concludes Chapter 1, which has presented an overview of this dissertation, the aims and scope of this research, definitions of terms and key concepts relevant to this research, as well as providing an introduction to Falun Gong and its many relevant descriptions. Chapter 1 has also presented the theoretical framework for this research, which is based on the link between spirituality/ religion and health. It presents the primary and secondary aims of this research, which is to investigate the health-wellness effects of Falun Gong as perceived by individuals who practice Falun Gong and to obtain an international demographic profile of Falun Gong practitioners respectively. This is the first doctoral research that involves a comparison group and investigates whether individuals who practice Falun Gong experience better health-wellness than those who do not.

This Australian-based research will indicate that individuals who practice Falun Gong experience better health-wellness outcomes than those who do not. Findings from this research will provide insight into and knowledge of the health-wellness effects of Falun Gong, its use as a mind-body self-improvement cultivation technique, its potential as an adjunct to counseling, and in health-wellness promotion. The findings and recommendations are pertinent to all readers, researchers, members of the public, and all health professionals, seeking to learn more about the health-wellness effects of Falun Gong and how to be better equipped to help individuals who practice Falun Gong and other mind-body spiritual meditation techniques for self-care, mind-body, and spiritual self-improvement. Readers are once again encouraged to read this dissertation with "a new manner of seeing" (Plotinus, 1975, p. 42), as suggested in the opening chapter quotation from the Greek philosopher, Plotinus.

Chapter 2 now presents the literature review.

CHAPTER 2

Literature Review

In fact, let me tell everyone that matter and mind are one thing.
(H. Li, 2001b, p. 28)

Conventional medicine will keep breaking new ground in treatment and prevention, yet often the most effective solutions are found in the medicine cabinet of the mind. (Oz, 2003, p. 2)

2.1 Chapter overview

This chapter presents a comprehensive review and critical analysis of studies and literature relating to this health-wellness research on Falun Gong. It covers the historical contexts, trends in meditative practices, role and effects of meditation (in the helping professions), and related literature. A review of the literature exploring the link between spirituality/religion and health is also included, as it forms the theoretical framework for this research.

Despite the growing interest in and awareness of Eastern mind-body practices, there is a dearth of research investigating the health-wellness effects of Falun Gong. There are numerous articles, books, and several academic and postgraduate studies conducted on Falun Gong, such as Bruseker (2000), Lowe (2003), Ownby (2003b; 2008a), Porter (2003; 2005) and S. J. Palmer (2003), but the focus was not on health-wellness effects. Therefore, a literature review in its broader context had to be conducted for this research. Meditation and other similar Eastern spiritual "meditative movement" (C. E. Rogers et al., 2009, p. 246) practices, such as yoga, tai chi, and qigong, were also included.

2.2 Aim, objective, and scope of the literature review

The aim of this review is to examine literature relating to the health-wellness effects of Falun Gong practice. However, a lack of evidence-based literature on the health-wellness effects of Falun Gong practice required literature and evidence on meditation and similar practices for comparison. Hence the scope of the review for this chapter focuses on meditation and non-Falun Gong literature that explores other similar kinds of meditative practice. The objective is to ascertain whether these other mind-body, self-improvement and self-help meditative practices (similar to Falun Gong) are effective in improving and maintaining health and wellness.

The literature review in this chapter broadly comprises the following:
- Historical contexts and trends in meditative/spiritual practices;
- Role of meditation in the helping professions;
- Effects of meditation on health;
- Other effects of meditation;
- Effects of yoga on health;
- Effects of tai chi on health;
- Effects of qigong on health; and
- Link between spirituality/religion and health.

The review commenced in late 2003 when this doctoral research project first began. Search inclusion criteria were Falun Gong, its health and wellness effects, role and effects of meditation, in English language only from the 1970s to the current time. Christian meditation was excluded to narrow the scope of review to Eastern meditative and spiritual practices. Literature on the link between spirituality/religion and health were also included. Data bases used comprised Academic Elite, Academic Search Premier, Blackwell Synergy, EbscoHost, CINAHL, Health source nursing/academic edition, Medline, PsycArticles, PsycINFO, Psychology and Behavioral Sciences Collection, Religion and Philosophy Collection, SAGE full-text collection, ScienceDirect, Social sciences citations index, Wiley interscience, and The Cochrane Collaboration. Falun Gong websites were accessed via Internet search engines and email contacts with other researchers, and journalist-writers were also utilized.

Key words and terms such as meditation, benefits of meditation, meditation and stress, meditation and wellness, wellness counseling, spirituality and wellness, religion and health, and spirituality and health were used after searches for Falun Gong or Falun Dafa and health, on Academic Search Premier, PsycArticles, PsycINFO, religion and philosophy yielded no results. Search subjects were then widened to include other meditative practices, such as Vipassana meditation, mindfulness meditation, yoga, tai chi, and qigong, with complementary and alternative medicine (CAM), Mind-Body Medicine (MBM), mind-body therapies, and mind-body techniques added later. English language journals, magazines, newspapers articles, websites, books, and reports, including unpublished works, were also sourced and reviewed for content and relevance.

Three decisions were made during the literature search. The first decision was to use the term Falun Gong instead of Falun Dafa in this dissertation. Falun Gong seems to be more widely used, as indicated during the literature searches. The second decision was to widen the scope of the literature review, to include other similar spiritual, "meditative movement" (C. E. Rogers et al., 2009, p. 246) practices because of the lack of evidence-based studies on the health-wellness effects of Falun Gong. The term 'meditative movement' has been recently ascribed to mind-body practices that combine breathing techniques, gentle physical movements or postures with meditation, such as yoga, qigong, and tai chi (C. E. Rogers et al., 2009). The third decision was to choose the Internet survey method and the Short Form (SF-36) Health Survey (Ware Jr., 2008; Ware Jr. & Sherbourne, 1992) for research data gathering for consistency and ease of administration as confirmed by the review.

2.3 Historical contexts and trends in meditative/ spiritual practices

Walsh (1989) noted that numerous clinical studies on meditation indicated the effectiveness and the wide-ranging benefits of ancient Eastern meditative practices that dated back nearly 3000 years: "Until recently very little was known of these practices in the West, and what was known was frequently misunderstood and dismissed" (Walsh, 1989, p. 548).

These Eastern meditative and spiritual practices have been described as "Eastern psychologies" (Fadiman & Frager, 1994, p. 503), "Asian psychotherapies," "Asian psychologies" or "Asian psychology" (Goleman, 1976, p. 42; Walsh, 1989, p. 547), or "esoteric traditions" (Carpenter, 1977, p. 394). Others considered meditation as the "royal road to the transpersonal" (Walsh & Vaughan, 1993, p. 47) and a technique for transcending, or "going beyond the individual or personal to encompass wider aspects of humankind, life, psyche and cosmos" (Walsh & Vaughan, 1993, p. 3). These are significant claims about the potential of meditative practices taking individuals beyond their being, based on their belief and practice rather than evidence, and show the impact these practices seem to have had.

Over the past two decades, an increasing number of individuals in developed countries have been turning to Eastern meditative spiritual practices (Atwood & Maltin, 1991; Delmonte, 1984; Easton, 2005; Krisanaprakornkit et al., 2006; Monk-Turner, 2003; Shapiro Jr., 1980; Singer, 2006; Walsh, 1989; Walsh & Vaughan, 1993). Monk-Turner (2003), reported that according to estimated figures from the World Health Organization (WHO), about 65% to 80% of the global population resort to traditional or alternative medicine, which indicates its appeal and presumed effectiveness.

Many therapists, counselors, other health professionals, and researchers recognized the therapeutic potential and other wide-ranging benefits of Eastern meditative practices and began exploring ways to integrate meditation with therapy (Atwood & Maltin, 1991; Bogart, 1991; Carpenter, 1977; Easton, 2005; Goleman, 1976; Marlatt & Kristeller, 1999; McCown, 2004; Ospina. et al., 2008; Perez-De-Albeniz & , 2000; Schopen & Freeman, 1992; Singer, 2006; Walsh, 1989; Walsh & Vaughan, 1993). Shapiro, Jr. (1980), presented a comprehensive exploration of different aspects of meditation, including clinical and psychotherapeutic uses and issues with meditation research methodologies. Shapiro, Jr. (1980), considered meditation a self-regulation strategy, a self-help, self-improvement, and self-care practice that enabled individuals to address their own personal needs for physical and emotional health and wellness.

Different authors noted the emerging trend of Eastern meditative and spiritual practices as being more readily accepted in the West (Carpenter, 1977; Cowen & Adams, 2005; Shapiro Jr., 1980; Walsh & Vaughan, 1993) for various reasons. Most individuals seemed to turn to meditation and other mind-body therapies, not because of their dissatisfaction with conventional medicine, but because these practices corresponded with their values, beliefs and attitudes for a healthy, wellness lifestyle (Astin, 1998; Gordon & Edwards, 2005; Wu et al., 2007).

The different reasons for Western researchers, counselors, other health care professionals, and various individuals being drawn to meditation include:

- Accounts of the extraordinary effects of meditation;
- Stories of altered states of consciousness by Eastern meditation masters;
- Meditation as an integral part in transpersonal development and transpersonal psychology/counseling;
- Frustration of health care professionals with mainstream medicine and their search for non-drug-related self-regulation intervention strategies;
- A changing focus from an illness approach to the wellness model of health;
- Clients/patients seeking alternative solutions and expressing openness to adopt a more proactive and holistic approach to their health issues;
- Economic considerations, as many spiritual meditative practices are either free or less costly than conventional medical care;
- Less invasive and fewer side effects than conventional medicine;
- Wide-ranging psycho-physiological effects of meditation;
- Meditation as a mental exercise for the brain, assisting in the promotion of positive emotions, well-being, and happiness; and
- Mind-body benefits of meditation, such as equanimity, tranquility, joy, and peace, which is increasingly being sought by individuals in their busy lifestyles (Carlson, Ursuliak, Goodey, Angeen, & Speca, 2001; Easton, 2005; Gordon & Edwards, 2005; Monk-Turner, 2003; Naranjo & Ornstein, 1971; S. J. Palmer, 2003; Shapiro Jr., 1980, pp. 3-4; Walsh, 1989; Walsh & Vaughan, 1993).

Considerable literature indicated the popularity and increasing use of CAM, mind-body therapies, Eastern meditative and spiritual practices in Australia, the United States, and elsewhere (Barnes, Powell-Griner, McFann, & Nahin,

2004; Bishop & Lewith, 2008; Eisenberg et al., 1998; Kessler et al., 2001; M. M. Lee, Lin, Wrensch, Adler, & Eisenberg, 2000; Long, Huntley, & Ernst, 2001; Mamtani & Cimino, 2002; Mehta, Phillips, Davis, & McCarthy, 2007; Monk-Turner, 2003; Shorofi & Arbon, 2009; Siti et al., 2009; Upchurch et al., 2007; Peter M. Wolsko, Eisenberg, Davis, Ettner, & Phillips, 2002; Peter M Wolsko et al., 2004; Yeh, Davis, & Phillips, 2006). Findings from the 2002 US National Health Interview Survey (NHIS) showed 62% of adult Americans resorting to CAM use over a 12-month period (Barnes et al., 2004; Mehta et al., 2007). A study conducted in Adelaide (South Australia) on patients in four hospitals indicated that CAM use is prevalent among hospitalized patients: 90% of patients reported CAM use, although most of them did not inform their doctors or nurses (Shorofi & Arbon, 2009).

According to the South Australian study and the 2002 NHIS survey, more women than men reported using CAM (Barnes et al., 2004; Shorofi & Arbon, 2009), with 57% of women reporting CAM use in the Australian study (Shorofi & Arbon, 2009). Forty percent of American women had used CAM therapies (Upchurch et al., 2007), as did more educated Asian American women (Mehta et al., 2007). Findings from another survey on CAM use among women with depression showed that 54% of these women reported using CAM therapies (Wu et al., 2007). Two most popular reasons for CAM use among women were the benefit of combining CAM with conventional treatment (54.4%) and that it would be "interesting to try" (52%) (Upchurch et al., 2007, p. 107).

Meditation and yoga were listed as the ten most popular CAM, mind-body therapies during the 12-month period in the 2002 NHIS survey (Barnes et al., 2004). Their popularity persisted as an indication of more individuals taking control and seeking a more proactive approach to health and wellness maintenance (Barnes et al., 2004; Carlson et al., 2001; Gordon & Edwards, 2005; Ospina et al., 2008; Upchurch et al., 2007; Peter M. Wolsko et al., 2004; Yeh et al., 2006). Other writers, like Lindberg (2005), conducted a comprehensive review of studies focusing on the management of chronic ailments and the beneficial effects of meditation and spirituality on older adults. This review, which included studies over the past 25 years, indicated that meditation could help ease anxiety, lessen despair, offer hope and enhance self-esteem for older adults living in nursing homes (Lindberg, 2005). A simple, low cost, or free meditative practice can thus provide solace, enhance mind-body health-wellness, and promote positive ageing—something that drugs try to do with higher costs and undesirable side effects.

Another team of researchers, recognizing that meditation can help promote health and wellness, conducted a systematic and comprehensive review of 400 clinical trials from 1956 to 2005 (Ospina et al., 2008). Their review focused on five varieties of meditative practices used in health care, including mindfulness meditation, yoga, tai chi, and qigong (Ospina et al., 2008), and examined the methodological characteristics. Their findings indicated that most randomized controlled trials (RCT) on meditative practices were compromised, although their quality was found to improve significantly over time (Ospina et al., 2008).

Considerations of meditation for this literature review included Falun Gong, Vipassana (mindfulness meditation), Transcendental Meditation (TM), and meditative movement practices like yoga, tai chi, and qigong. Falun Gong is similar to other meditative movement practices in that its exercise movements are slow, rhythmic, meditative, and performed with practice instruction music (H. Li, 2001a). The effects of these meditative practices will be reviewed and discussed in separate sections in this chapter.

2.4 Role of meditation in the helping professions

This section discusses literature exploring the role of meditation and its application as an adjunct or therapeutic intervention in psychotherapy, counseling, and other health care services. An increasing number of therapists, counselors, and others in the health care professions readily integrate meditation into their counseling and psychotherapeutic practices (Atwood & Maltin, 1991; Bogart, 1991; Carpenter, 1977; Goldberg, 1982; Goleman, 1976; Marlatt & Kristeller, 1999; Schopen & Freeman, 1992; Singer, 2006; Walsh, 1989; Walsh & Bugental, 2005). In 1977, the American Psychological Association (APA) developed a position statement on meditation, recognizing the supporting and beneficial role of meditation in the therapeutic process (Schopen & Freeman, 1992, p. 5; Singer, 2006, p. 3). Delmonte (1985) noted that by the 1980s, meditation was widely used as an adjunct to counseling and psychotherapy in the West. Despite APA's recognition and continuing interest, the use of meditation in counseling and psychotherapy remains peripheral and not a mainstream practice (Singer, 2006).

Bogart (1991) also recognized the escalating interest in meditation as an adjunct to counseling and psychotherapy, and evaluated studies exploring the application and relevance of meditation in Western helping professions. He evaluated the pros and cons of meditation, its benefits, relevance, implications, considerations, and the potential risks of the use of meditation in the helping professions (Bogart, 1991). While Jungian and psychoanalytic therapists challenged the use of meditation, claiming it as regressive, encouraging dissociation, and ignoring the unconscious, transpersonal therapists argued in favor of meditation (Bogart, 1991). The latter believed the effects of meditation were encompassing and far outweighed any perceived notions against its integration into psychotherapy and counseling practices (Bogart, 1991).

Walsh and Vaughan (1993) discussed how meditation could "complement and catalyze therapy" (p. 55) for both the therapist and the client:

> In addition to cultivating healthy qualities such as calm and equanimity, it can enhance empathy and provide insight into mental processes and the origins of pathology. On the theoretical side, meditation practice and research offer insights into the nature of mind, maturation, and transpersonal experiences (Walsh & Vaughan, 1993, p. 55).

The clinical use of meditation in the helping professions pioneered in the 1970s, with researchers focusing on the effects and implications of meditation in the management of anxiety, stress, and psychological distress (Marlatt & Kristeller, 1999). Marlatt and Kristeller (1999) examined the role of meditation in therapeutic settings, offering specific uses of meditation as a "global method of stress management, relaxation, and personal centering" (p. 74). They proposed meditation as a way to "attain a balanced lifestyle" (p. 74) and to create harmony in one's daily life (Marlatt & Kristeller, 1999). Carpenter (1977) discussed the use of meditation in clinical and therapeutic settings, and noted that Buddhism, with its emphasis on compassion, was the "direct inspiration for many of the applications of meditative components to modern psychotherapy" (p. 395). Goleman (1976) also noted that many researchers examined the clinical use of meditation. He posited that meditation for health and wellness may not be ideal for everyone, and hence may be unsuitable for mental health patients, individuals with schizoid personalities, acute emotional problems, and obsessive-compulsive behaviors (Goleman, 1976) as they may not have the mental prowess to practice it.

Schopen and Freeman (1992) presented a different view that meditation could even substitute "counseling as a healing force or change agent for certain clients" (p. 5). They described meditation as a "meta-therapy" (p. 5) that induces relaxation, minimizes stress and tension, supports insights gained from talk therapy, and as a self-help technique for clients in between appointments (Schopen & Freeman, 1992). Like Goleman (1976), Schopen and Freeman (1992) cautioned that meditation should be incorporated into therapy with professional care and advised against using it with severely disturbed clients.

In other words, like other CAM, MBM, or mind-body therapies, meditation has contraindications and might not be suitable for everyone (Goldberg, 1982; Goleman, 1976; Schopen & Freeman, 1992). This is because meditation requires mental activity or mind cultivation. This is the same with Falun Gong because Falun Gong cultivates the mind, or specifically the main consciousness, and hence is unsuitable for individuals with delusions, hallucinations, and severe distortions in perceptions of reality, and those with serious mental disorders, such as schizophrenia, mania or psychosis. Mr. Li Hongzhi (2001b) explained that psychosis occurred because one's main consciousness becomes weak and loses its ability to take charge of the person: "It is always in a daze and cannot become conscious" (2001b, p. 219), hence rendering the individual unable to practice meditation.

Jacobs (2001) noted that meditation and various mind-body practices were used in conjunction with conventional medicine rather than as an alternative. Medical professionals like Mehmet Oz (2003), cardiovascular surgeon and director of the Cardiovascular Institute, Columbia University Medical Center in New York, U.S., integrated meditation with surgical intervention, using meditation to help prepare patients for surgery and to assist them in post-surgery recovery and healing. "Why? Because it works" (Oz, 2003, p. 1). The best therapeutic intervention resided in the "medicine cabinet of the mind"

(Oz, 2003, p. 2). He explained the benefits of meditation, identifying one study on meditation where a 15-minute meditation twice a day could lessen medical visits over a six-month period with a health care saving of US$200 per person (Oz, 2003, p. 2).

2.5 Effects of meditation on health

There is considerable literature supporting the health-wellness benefits of meditation and a plethora of studies exploring the effects of meditation dating from the 1970s to the present (A. Chiesa & Serretti, 2009; Goldberg, 1982; Grossman, Niemann, Schmidt, & Walach, 2004; Kang, Choi, & Ryu, 2009; Lazar et al., 2005; McCown, 2004; Monk-Turner, 2003; Perez-De-Albeniz & Holmes, 2000; Schreiner & Malcolm, 2008; Schwartz, Davidson, & Goleman, 1978; Sumter, Monk-Turner, & Turner, 2009; Tanner et al., 2009; Walsh & Bugental, 2005). Different studies investigated the use and effects of meditation on different conditions, such as anxiety (Delmonte, 1985; Goldberg, 1982; Gross et al., 2009; Kang et al., 2009; Krisanaprakornkit et al., 2006; Miller, Fletcher, & Kabat-Zinn, 1995; Schwartz et al., 1978; Tacón, McComb, Caldera, & Randolph, 2003), attention deficit hyperactivity disorder (ADHD) (Krisanaprakornkit, C., & N., 2007; Zylowska et al., 2008), depression (Gross et al., 2009; Scherer-Dickson, 2004; Schreiner & Malcolm, 2008; Selhub, 2007; Teasdale et al., 2000), stress management (Carlson et al., 2001; A. Chiesa & Serretti, 2009; Kang et al., 2009; Shapiro, Schwartz, & Bonner, 1998; Speca, Carlson, Goodey, & Angeen, 2000), post-traumatic stress disorder (PTSD) (Brooks & Scarano, 1985), and positive self-concept (Emavardhana & Tori, 1997). Other studies examined the effects of meditation on the quality of life (Carlson, Speca, Patel, & Faris, 2007; Jayadevappa et al., 2007; Reibel, Greeson, Brainard, & Rosenzweig, 2001; Roth & Robbins, 2004), and in educational (Christopher, Christopher, Dunnagan, & Schure, 2006; Kang et al., 2009; Laselle & Russell, 1993; Schure, Christopher, & Christopher, 2008) and correctional settings (Sumter, Monk-Turner, & Turner, 2007; Sumter et al., 2009). These studies reflected the potential diversity in the use of meditation for health and wellness, and provided insight into the possible uses of meditation for varying conditions and settings.

In a comprehensive review of 75 scientific papers from the Medline and Psychlit databases, ranging from 1989 to June 1999, Perez-De-Albeniz and Holmes (2000) provided a summary of the physiological, behavioral and psychological effects of meditation which included:

- Increased positive emotions, such as happiness and joy;
- Increased positive thoughts;
- Improved problem-solving skills;
- Improved self-confidence;
- Improved memory;
- Enhanced self-awareness;
- Enhanced acceptance, compassion, and tolerance towards self and others;
- Better relaxation, resilience, and ability to self-regulate emotions;
- Improvement in psychological well-being;
- Decreased anxiety;
- Decreased substance abuse;
- Hormonal and metabolic effects or changes; and
- Lower heart rate and blood pressure, and better muscle relaxation (Perez-De-Albeniz & Holmes, 2000, pp. 2, 3).

Perez-De-Albeniz and Holmes (2000) reported wide-ranging psychological and physiological effects of meditation, but also articulated that none of these findings were based on "properly randomized and controlled trials" (Perez-De-Albeniz & Holmes, 2000, p. 2). This raises a paradox in research where specific individualistic effects may not be 'proven' through empirical studies, but can be soundly verified through qualitative studies.

Monk-Turner (2003) discussed the mind-body connection of meditation as well as the psycho-physiological and spiritual benefits of meditation, citing writers, researchers and advocates of meditation, such as: Joan Borysenko (1987), author of the book *Minding the body, mending the mind*; Dr. Herbert Benson (1975, 1996), originator of the 'Relaxation Response' model (Crombie, 2002; G. D. Jacobs, 2001); and Kabat-Zinn (1990), who developed the mindfulness-based stress reduction (MBSR) program at the Stress Reduction Clinic of the University of Massachusetts Medical Center (Shapiro et al., 1998). Monk-Turner (2003) alluded to different studies on meditation to illustrate its wide-ranging benefits, such as stress reduction, enhanced happiness, well-being, and self-confidence, a reduction in the use of tranquillizers, other drugs, and medical services, including reduction of aggression and violence in prison settings, and recidivism upon release. Meditation was found to reduce stress, enhance self-confidence, boost levels of happiness for the incarcerated population, and hence could be a cost-effective intervention strategy for inmates and staff in correctional settings (Sumter et al., 2007, 2009).

Delmonte (1985) specifically reviewed studies on the use of meditation in anxiety management and found that frequent and consistent meditation practice seemed to help lower anxiety, although there was no strong empirical data to verify that meditation was more effective than other relaxation techniques. A Cochrane systematic review of randomized controlled trials (RCT) on meditation for anxiety disorders could not make any definitive inference about the effects of meditation due to a limited number of studies (Krisanaprakornkit et al., 2006).

Transcendental Meditation (TM) was found to be a beneficial adjunctive modality for post-traumatic stress disorder (PTSD) in Vietnam war veterans in one RCT (Brooks & Scarano, 1985). Another RCT on TM as an adjunct to conventional treatment for cardiovascular illness indicated that TM helped to lower stress and significantly improve the quality of life of heart patients (Jayadevappa et al., 2007). According to the official TM website, there are hundreds of evidence-based research studies that indicated TM to be beneficial for stress and anxiety, brain function, and cardiovascular health (www.tm.org).

There are numerous evidence-based studies on mindfulness meditation (also known as Vipassana meditation) (Marlatt & Kristeller, 1999), and especially on the MBSR program (Carlson et al., 2007; Grossman et al., 2004; Miller et al., 1995; Reibel et al., 2001; Schure et al., 2008; Shapiro et al., 1998; Tacón et al., 2003). MBSR is described as a hospital-based, patient-focused, clinical and wellness group intervention stress reduction program that combines mindfulness meditation, yoga and relaxation techniques to teach patients with chronic medical conditions alternative ways of living a healthier and better quality life (Carlson et al., 2007; Christopher et al., 2006; Reibel et al., 2001; Tacón et al., 2003).

These studies investigated the effects of mindfulness meditation on specific conditions, ranging from anxiety disorders (Kang et al., 2009; Krisanaprakornkit et al., 2006; Miller et al., 1995; Tacón et al., 2003), attention deficit hyperactivity disorder (ADHD) (Krisanaprakornkit et al., 2007; Zylowska et al., 2008), brain and immune function (Davidson et al., 2003) chronic pain (Rosenzweig et al., 2009; Zeidan, Gordon, Merchant, & Goolkasian, 2009), depression (Scherer-Dickson, 2004; Schreiner & Malcolm, 2008; Selhub, 2007; Teasdale et al., 2000), stress reduction (Carlson et al., 2001; Kang et al., 2009; Shapiro et al., 1998; Speca et al., 2000), and quality of life (Bedard et al., 2003; Carlson et al., 2007; Reibel et al., 2001; Roth & Robbins, 2004). Their findings indicated beneficial effects of MBSR and supported its use for different presenting conditions.

Other researchers discussed the relevance of teaching meditation, such as MBSR, and its use as a self-care practice in counselor training programs (Christopher et al., 2006; Schure et al., 2008). Due to the demands and nature of their work, counselors and other health care professionals are often susceptible to stress and emotional exhaustion, and hence there is a need for the provision of self-care techniques during their training (Schure et al., 2008; Shapiro, Astin, Bishop, & Cordova, 2005). Shapiro, Schwartz and Bonner (1998) evaluated the effects of MBRS on premedical and medical students, and found it helped to reduce state and trait anxiety, overall psychological distress, and depression. Another RCT also indicated beneficial effects of MBSR, such as stress reduction, enhanced quality of life, and self-compassion in health care professionals (Shapiro et al., 2005).

While there were studies conducted on undergraduate, nursing, and medical students, Christopher et al. (2006) noted that there were no published studies investigating the use of mindfulness meditation in counseling curricula and students. Subsequently Schure et al. (2008) conducted a four-year qualitative study investigating the effect of teaching yoga, meditation, and qigong to counseling students and discovered these meditative practices had beneficial effects on the students, as well as on their counseling skills and therapeutic relationships.

2.5.1 Other effects of meditation

Literature illustrating other effects of meditation included increased plasma melatonin levels (Tooley, Armstrong, Norman, & Sali, 2000), higher dopamine levels (Kjaer et al., 2002), changes in brain and immune function (Davidson et al., 2003) changes in body temperature (Crombie, 2002), enhanced positive emotions of happiness, joy, and well-being (Easton, 2005; Fredrickson, 2000; Lemonick, 2005; Wallis, 2005), and brain plasticity or changes in brain structure (Lazar et al., 2005) Regular and ongoing meditation was linked with increased cortical thickness of the brain and thus may delay the ageing process (Lazar et al., 2005)

Marlatt and Kristeller (1999) outlined five categories of therapeutic components or effects of meditation. These five categories were: deep physiological relaxation state; altered consciousness, brain and neurological functioning; a form of "positive addiction"; state of heightened mindful awareness or meta-cognitive practice; and meditation as a spiritual discipline (Marlatt & Kristeller, 1999, pp. 72-74).

While most studies on meditation reported positive and beneficial effects of meditation, some unpleasant effects were found (Bogart, 1991; Goldberg, 1982). Perez-De-Albeniz and Holmes (2000) summarized some of the side effects of meditation, which included boredom, pain, uncomfortable mind-body sensations, meditation-induced anxiety and tension, confusion, a "spaced out" feeling, and other negative emotions, such as fear, anger, and sadness (p. 51). They cited Shapiro Jr. (1992, 1994) on the topic of contraindications and adverse effects of meditation (Perez-De-Albeniz & Holmes, 2000). Shapiro Jr. (also cited in Perez-De-Albeniz & Holmes, 2000; Shapiro Jr., 1992) reported that the length of practice made no difference to the characteristics of the side effects and that 63% of respondents (n=27) attending a Vipassana meditation retreat experienced at least one unpleasant effect, while about seven percent had acute negative effects. This finding should be interpreted with caution and within context. Another researcher stated that Vipassana meditation retreats involved "up to 10 days of intensive meditation, several hours per day, and other strict observances, such as not talking and encouragement to maintain strict postures for long periods of time" (Manocha, 2000, p. 1137), unlike a 15-minute or 30-minute meditation session at home, or in a pleasant therapeutic or clinical setting, and hence would be physically and psychologically demanding even for an experienced meditator.

There is also a disparity in the therapeutic effects of meditation between novice and experienced meditators, as there are short-term and long-term benefits (Goldberg, 1982) Goldberg (1982) stated that negative outcomes in meditation studies could be due to a fleeting encounter with the practice, lack of meditation experience, or respondents merely emulating the technique and not congruently engaging in the meditation practice. He made the analogy of the difference in therapeutic effects between a beginner and an experienced meditator with that of a novice musician and a virtuoso (Goldberg, 1982).

2.5.2 Concepts relating to the effects of meditation

The following subsections briefly explain two concepts that support and explain the effects and benefits of meditation. The first is the Relaxation Response (RR) (Crombie, 2002; G. D. Jacobs, 2001) and the second refers to the principle of Reciprocal Inhibition (RI) (Goleman, 1976).

2.5.2.1 Relaxation Response

It is noted that meditation involves mental activity that elicits a deep physical relaxation state, described as a "wakeful hypometabolic state" (Marlatt & Kristeller, 1999, p. 72) or a state of "relaxed wakefulness" (Bogart, 1991, p. 4). Dr. Herbert Benson, pioneer in Mind-Body Medicine and Associate Professor of Medicine at the Harvard Medical School, coined the term 'Relaxation Response' (RR) to describe these therapeutic effects of meditation (Crombie, 2002; G. D. Jacobs, 2001). Benson explained that meditation produced a distinct "physiological state opposite to stress" (cited in Crombie, 2002, p. 2). Four prerequisites are required to elicit the RR: relaxed muscles; quiet ambience; calm mind or taking no notice of intrusive thoughts; and reciting "a word, sound, phrase or short prayer" (Crombie, 2002, p. 2; G. D. Jacobs, 2001, pp. S-88).

The RR elicited by meditation helps to lower and regulate blood pressure, metabolism, breathing, and heart rate (Crombie, 2002). It alleviates the "fight-or-flight response," also called the "stress response" (G. D. Jacobs, 2001, pp. S-84, S-85, & S-86). A unique characteristic of the RR is the noticeable reduction in the body's consumption of oxygen (Faneuli, 1997). Benson and his colleagues made use of the RR technique for anxiety, depression, anger management, high blood pressure, irregular heartbeat, insomnia, infertility, and also to relax "those traumatized by the deaths of others, or by diagnoses of cancer or other painful, life-threatening illnesses" (Crombie, 2002, p. 2). A one-year follow-up study indicated that the RR technique produced both short and long-term therapeutic benefits on sufferers of irritable bowel syndrome (Keefer & Blanchard, 2002).

2.5.2.2 Principle of Reciprocal Inhibition

The American Psychological Association (APA) *Dictionary of Psychology* defines the Principle of Reciprocal Inhibition (RI) as "a technique in behavior therapy that aims to replace an undesired response with a desired one" (VandenBos, 2007, p. 776). RI originated from U.S. psychologist Joseph Wolpe (1958) (cited in Bogart, 1991, p. 5; VandenBos, 2007), who postulated that a negative response could be removed by introducing an opposite and positive response. Bogart (1991), in referring to Goleman's (1976) study of the Abhidhamma Buddhist teachings, explained that RI, which forms the basis of contemporary behavioral self-regulation technique, can be used to replace or eliminate a negative emotion or unhealthy mental state with a healthy and positive response, like relaxation or meditation.

Goleman (1976) stated that "reciprocal inhibition of unhealthy mental factors by healthy ones" (p. 43) comprised the focal point of the Abhidhamma teachings for positive mental health. There are 14 unhealthy mental states, such as envy, egoism (self-centeredness), shamelessness, and worry (anxiety) in Abhidhamma teachings that can be replaced by 14 healthy mental states, which include insight, mindfulness, modesty, impartiality or non-attachment, and kindness or compassion (Goleman, 1976, pp. 43-44). According to the RI principle, meditation serves as the means to better health and wellness in which unhealthy mental states can be replaced by healthy ones such as joy, compassion, and contentment, through "self-regulation and retraining of attentional habits" (Goleman, 1976, p. 44).

However, the RR model and the RI principle are susceptible to criticisms. Bogart (1991) presented a comprehensive argument against them with criticisms, including: 1) RR does not explain the subjective meditation experience or process; 2) meditation elicits different effects on different individuals, or the same individuals at different times; 3) meditation may not decrease drug-induced anxiety by substituting relaxation or meditation for the drug; and 4) meditation is a dynamic process and different meditation techniques elicit different results. Despite these criticisms, the RR model and RI do help to explain the effects and benefits of meditation.

CHAPTER 3

Falun Gong-Related Literature Review

3.1 Chapter overview

This chapter focuses on the review of existing Falun Gong literature, its health and wellness effects. Due to a lack of literature and studies exploring the health and wellness effects of Falun Gong, this chapter also includes a broad literature review of other Eastern meditative practices, such as tai chi and qigong.

3.2 Demographic profile of Falun Gong practitioners

Studies on the demographic profile of Falun Gong practitioners can be placed into two categories: surveys in mainland China prior to the persecution of Falun Gong in July 1999; and studies of Falun Gong practitioners outside of China after July 1999. Several large-scale studies were conducted in different regions across mainland China: in Beijing (Author Unknown, 2002; Dan et al., 1998; Porter, 2003; Wang et al., 1998; Zhang & Xiao, 1996), Dalian region (Author Unknown, 1998, 2002; Porter, 2003), Guandong province and Wuhan (Author Unknown, 2002). Table 3.1 shows the frequency and gender distribution of Falun Gong respondents from these studies.

Table 3.1 Gender distribution of respondents from mainland China health survey

Place	Frequency	Male	Female
Guangdong Province	12,553	3,502	9,051
Beijing	12,731	3,554	9,177
Wuhan	2,005	563	1,442
Dalian Region	6,478	1,501	4,977
Zizhu Park, Beijing	584	174	410
Total	34,351	9,294	25,057

Source: (Author Unknown, 2002)

According to the "Summary of health surveys conducted in mainland China to assess Falun Gong's effects on healing illness and maintaining fitness" (Author Unknown, 2002), there were more female (73%, n=25,057) than male respondents (27%, n=9,294), and over 62% of total respondents (n=34,351) were more than 50 years old. These surveys also indicated that mainland Chinese practitioners came from all walks of life (Author Unknown, 2002; Zhang & Xiao, 1996), and "included men and women, rich and poor, educated and uneducated, powerful and powerless, urban and rural, Party and non-Party" (Ownby, 2003b, p. 305).

The demographic profile of Falun Gong practitioners outside of China came from studies conducted in Canada and the United States (Burgdoff, 2003; Lowe, 2003; Ownby, 2003b, 2008a; S. J. Palmer, 2003; Porter, 2003, 2005). Burgdoff's (2003) participant-observer field study indicated that about 90% of Falun Gong practitioners in Columbus, Ohio (U.S.), were ethnically Chinese. Lowe's (2003) US-based Internet survey showed that 98% of Falun Gong respondents (n=83) were "well-educated Chinese intellectuals in most American, Canadian, and (to a less [sic] extent) European university towns" (p. 268). S. J. Palmer (2003) and Ownby (2003b; 2008a) initiated field studies using self-designed questionnaires and face-to-face interviews with Falun Gong practitioners in Montreal, Ottawa, and Toronto (Canada), New York, Waco, and Dallas, Texas (U.S.).

The majority of North American Falun Gong practitioners were Chinese, female, married, well educated, financially wealthy, and younger (average age=40 years) than practitioners in mainland China (Ownby, 2001, 2003b, 2008a; S. J. Palmer, 2003). According to Ownby (2003b), Falun Gong "remains unabashedly Chinese" and is "overwhelmingly Chinese (about 90% in North America)" (p. 308). He stated that "the average Chinese (Falun Gong) practitioner in North America is young, urban, dynamic, a successful recent immigrant largely living the American dream" (Ownby, 2008a, p. 138). Ownby (2003b) described Falun Gong practiced by Chinese in Canada as a "bourgeois movement" and that "the stereotypical practitioner lives in the suburbs and drives a Ford Taurus to her job in computers or finance" (p. 312).

Porter's (2003) master's thesis, *"Falun Gong in the United States: An ethnographic study,"* provided an insightful demographic profile of U.S. Falun Gong practitioners. His field study focused on the nature of Falun Gong practice, demographics, activities of practitioners, role of contact persons, and 'professional' practitioners such as nuns and monks residing in temples (Porter, 2003, 2005). North American practitioners were younger than mainland China Falun Gong practitioners, with 62% of them below 39 years of age (Porter, 2003). He also tabulated all existing studies on Falun Gong practitioners by their gender, age groups, ethnicity/nationality, level of education, and occupations (Porter, 2003, pp. 113-116). Table 3.2 shows a summary of the demographic profile of Falun Gong practitioners in mainland China and North America from existing studies.

Table 3.2 Demographic profile of Falun Gong practitioners from existing studies

Name/ Year	Study	Study Size	Gender	Age Range	Ethnicity/ Birth Country
1996	Beijing, China	355	F: 72%, 255 M: 28%,100	-	MC
1998 China	ZiZhu, Beijing	584	F: 30%, 174 M: 70%, 410	7-20: 2.2% 21-50: 29%,167	MC
1998	Guandong, China	12,553	F: 72%, 9,051 M: 28%, 3,502	<50: 49%, 6,076 >50: 51%, 6,433	MC
1998	Beijing, China	12,731	F: 72%, 9,177 M: 28%, 3,354	<10: 0.3%, 44 11-20: 1.4%, 176 21-30: 4.8%, 608 31-40: 8.4%, 1,071 41-50: 17.6%, 2,241 51-60: 27.5%, 3,498 >60: 40%, 5,093	MC
1998	Dalian, China	6,478	F: 77%, 4,977 M: 23%, 1501	<50: 29%, 1,864 >50: 71%, 4,614	MC
1998	Wuhan, China	2,005	F: 72%, 1,442 M: 28%, 563	<50: 38%, 768 >50: 62%, 1,237	MC
Ownby & Palmer 2001	Canada & US	78	F: 56%, 44 M: 44%, 34	Mean: 41.88 Median: 37	Chinese: 91%, 71 Westerners: 9%, 7
Lowe 2000	Internet	85	-	-	MC: 53%, 45; SIN: 35%, 30; M'sia: 10%, 8; US: 1%, 1; Rom: 1%, 1
Bourdoff 2001	Ohio, US	20-25	-	-	Chinese: 85-90%; 3-4 Westerners
Porter 2003	Tampa, Florida; Washing-ton DC, US	53	F: 22 (42%) M: 31 (58%)	Mean: 37.38 Median: 36 sd = 10.52 20-29: 14 (26%) 30-39: 19 (36%) 40-49: 11 (21%) 50-60: 9 (17%)	US born: 18 (34%) China born: 24 (45.3%) Taiwan born: 5 (9.4%) Elsewhere: 6 (11.3%)

MC: Mainland Chinese; M'sia: Malaysia; ROM: Romania; SIN: Singapore;
F: Female; M: Male
Source: (Authors Unknown, 1999; Porter, 2003, pp. 113-114)

Findings from another survey (not included in Table 3.2) on Canadian and U.S. Falun Gong practitioners indicated that 97% of respondents were ethnically

Chinese, that they were young and well educated, with the majority of them in computer information technology professions (Authors Unknown, 1999, 2003a). The survey indicated that the average length of practice was 26.4 months (sd=14.2) and that there were more female than male Falun Gong respondents, as shown in Table 3.3.

Table 3.3 Demographic profiles of Canadian and US Falun Gong practitioners

Year	Location of Study	Study Size	Gender (F=Female) (M=Male)	Age Range	Ethnicity/ Country of birth
1999-2000	Canada & US	235	F: 137 (58.3%) M: 98 (41%)	Mean: 38.9 sd = 13.6	Chinese: 137 (97%) Caucasian: 7 (3%)

Source: (Authors Unknown, 1999, 2003a)

3.3 Studies on the health-wellness effects of Falun Gong

Academic research on Falun Gong is still in its infancy (Penny, 2003), especially studies investigating health-wellness effects. This section reviews articles and existing studies that investigate the health effects of Falun Gong. Most of the health surveys were conducted in mainland China (Author Unknown, 1998, 2002; Dan et al., 1998; Wang et al., 1998; Zhang & Xiao, 1996) prior to the banning and persecution of Falun Gong in July 1999, in Taiwan (Authors Unknown, 2003b; Lio et al., 2003), and in North America (Authors Unknown, 1999, 2003a). However, there are concerns about the credibility, research rigor, and compliance with human research ethics regarding these studies. There is a lack of detailed information, transparency in documentation on the methodology, survey process, implementation, and systematic reporting of the findings of these surveys. Academics and researchers in the West have not readily accepted the results because of the absence of standards and rigor of research ethics that are comparable to Western universities. The anonymity of the authors and researchers for most of these studies and reports further diminishes credibility and accountability, especially for non–Falun Gong readers. From the Falun Gong practitioners' perspective, however, remaining anonymous is often done with the sincere intention to adhere to Falun Gong teachings in caring little for and not pursuing fame, self-interest and personal profit (H. Li, 2001b). Despite their limitations, these health surveys provided useful insights and information on the demographic profile of Falun Gong practitioners, health-wellness effects of Falun Gong, lifestyle and behavior modifications, and savings in medical and health care costs. To a certain extent, these surveys contributed to a benchmark for future studies investigating the healing potential and the health-wellness effects of Falun Gong.

Findings from the health surveys conducted in mainland China reported remarkable and positive effects of Falun Gong on health and wellness maintenance (Author Unknown, 1998, 2002; Clearwisdom editors, 2006; Dan et al., 1998; Life and hope renewed, 2005; McCoy & Zhang, n.d.; Wang et al., 1998; Zhang & Xiao, 1996). According to the "Summary of health surveys conducted in mainland China to assess Falun Gong's effects on healing illness and maintaining fitness" (Author Unknown, 2002), 83% of Falun Gong respondents reported full recovery from their illnesses, 16% reported health improvements, and one percent observed no changes to their health after commencing Falun Gong practice. The majority of respondents from the five surveys reported physical and mental health benefits, and eliminating their addictions to cigarette smoking, alcohol consumption, and gambling (Author Unknown, 2002). Findings from these studies are available on www.pureinsight.org, www.clearwisdom.net, and the Australian Falun Gong website, www.falunau.org/healthsurvey.htm. Although these surveys indicated significant health-wellness effects of Falun Gong and respondents' improvements in physical, mental, and psychological health and wellness after commencing Falun Gong practice, a lack of uniformity in methodology across the five surveys made consolidation of overall results difficult.

Besides highlighting the potential health-wellness effect of Falun Gong practice, these health surveys also indicated its medical and health cost-saving potential. Falun Gong respondents reported significant savings in health costs and medical expenses after starting Falun Gong practice (Dan et al., 1998; Life and hope renewed, 2005; Wang et al., 1998; Zhang & Xiao, 1996). See Table 3.4 for the average savings in medical and health care costs per person, and total savings in medical expenses in Chinese Yuan, the local currency in mainland China.

Table 3.4 Summary of savings in medical/health expenses

Location of Survey	Total Savings (Yuan)	Number of Respondents	Average Savings per Respondent
Beijing	41,700,000	12,731	3,270
Dailan	15,240,700	6,327	2,409
Guangdong	12,650,000	7,170	1,700
Total	69,590,700	26,228	2,653

Source: (Author Unknown, 2002, p. 6)

The monthly wage of the average worker in urban China was reported to be approximately 500 Yuan (Life and hope renewed, 2005, p. xii). Based on these findings, total medical cost savings from Falun Gong respondents was about 70 million Yuan per year, or 2,600 Yuan for each Falun Gong respondent before Falun Gong was banned in July 1999 and practitioners were persecuted by the CCP. The medical cost-saving potential was a substantial economic benefit for both the individual and the society.

Besides the mainland China health surveys, there were other Falun Gong health-wellness related studies from Taiwan (Authors Unknown, 2003b; Lio et al., 2003), United States (Authors Unknown, 1999, 2003a; Q. Li et al., 2005), and a single-case study from Australia (Lau, 2001). The Taiwan health survey indicated that Falun Gong helped to eliminate unhealthy and addictive lifestyle habits such as cigarette smoking, alcohol consumption, gambling, and chewing betel nuts (a common practice in Asian countries) (Authors Unknown, 2003b). Associate Professor Hu Yu-whuei, researcher at the National Taiwan University, stated that the Taiwan study indicated a decrease in medical expenses and about 50% reduction in the use of medical health insurance for Falun Gong respondents (Authors Unknown, 2003b). Hu, an expert in health economics, highlighted the potential for Falun Gong to promote health-wellness and save medical costs. She explained how Falun Gong could benefit the individual, society, and the country's medical health care system as a self-care practice and a health-wellness enhancing lifestyle (Authors Unknown, 2003b). Limitations of this brief report included lack of details on methodology, measures used, data collection, response rate, data analysis process, and the authors' names.

In an unpublished article on the Taiwan study, the participants' response rate was reported to be about 75% (Lio et al., 2003). This study used the SF-36 Health Survey and the SF-36 health scores of Taiwanese Falun Gong respondents, which were compared with Taiwan's SF-36 norm scores based on data from the 2001 Taiwan National Health Interview Survey (Lio et al., 2003, p. 8). Falun Gong respondents were found to be physically and mentally healthier than the general Taiwan population, and the health-wellness effects of Falun Gong increased with the years of practice, that is, the higher the number of years of practice, the better health, and the lower tendency to use medical care. To date, there is no published report of this Taiwan study in any peer-reviewed journal.

A North American health survey had results which were consistent with those from the other Falun Gong health surveys, with respondents reporting significant health improvements after starting Falun Gong practice (Authors Unknown, 1999, 2003a). Limitations of this health survey included unknown response rate, lack of study details, no systematic reporting of the entire research process, and anonymity of the researchers and writer(s) of the report (Authors Unknown, 1999, 2003a).

A phenomenological single-case study on the recovery from burnout of a U.S. health professional after commencing Falun Gong practice highlighted how Falun Gong offered an alternative coping strategy and helped buffer the negative effects of burnout (Lau, 2001). In another small-scale study involving Russian Falun Gong respondents, Professor Guluoji from the Russian Federal Internal Affairs Department reported a 75% health-wellness improvement rate in respondents (Author Unknown, 2003). An official statement affirming the potential for Falun Gong to promote health-wellness was issued, stating that Falun Gong "does not cause any danger or harm to human health and spirit" (Author Unknown, 2003, p. 1).

There were other Falun Gong studies conducted outside of mainland China indicating that the healing potential of Falun Gong and the promise of good health was what initially attracted many individuals to the practice (Lowe, 2003; Ownby, 2001, 2003a, 2003b, 2008a; S. J. Palmer, 2003; Porter, 2003). Falun Gong practice led to a health improvement for many Falun Gong respondents in Tampa and Washington, D.C. (U.S.) (Porter, 2003). Lowe's (2003) eight-question Internet survey revealed that the healing benefit of Falun Gong was one of the two most recurring responses to the question, "What first attracted you to Falun Dafa?" Likewise, Ownby's (2008a) study indicated "health benefits" was the third most frequent response as shown in Table 3.5.

Table 3.5 Results from Ownby's field study

No	What first attracted you to the practice?	Percent
1	Intellectual Content of Falun Gong teaching	28.9
2	Spiritual Growth/Elevation	26.6
3	Health Benefits	20.2
4	The Exercises	14.7
5	Master Li Hongzhi	7.3
6	The Community of Falun Gong practitioners	2.2

Source: (Ownby, 2008a, p. 141)

None of these studies were RCTs. The health surveys conducted in mainland China, Taiwan, Canada, and the U.S. lacked adequate information on the methodology and research process, transparency, and overall consistency. But this does not negate their relevance and importance, as the findings are still useful and relevant to this doctoral Falun Gong research, and in providing considerations for current and future Falun Gong health-wellness studies.

3.4 Evidence-based studies on Falun Gong

There is only one published peer-reviewed article of an evidence-based Falun Gong health study. A team of U.S. medical doctors and researchers conducted a pilot study on the effects of Falun Gong on gene expression and the role of neutrophils in Falun Gong practitioners (Q. Li et al., 2005). They investigated the effects of Falun Gong on the cellular and molecular levels of the human body using DNA micro-array technology (Q. Li et al., 2005). Respondents included six Asian Falun Gong practitioners with a control group of six healthy Asian non–Falun Gong individuals who did not engage in yoga, tai chi, qigong, or any other meditative movement practices. Superior gene expression, improved immunity, and longer lifespan of neutrophils were shown in Falun Gong respondents compared to the non–Falun Gong respondents (Q. Li et al., 2005). Falun Gong could influence gene expression, enhance immunity, balance metabolic rate, and promote cell regeneration on the basis of this study (Q. Li et al., 2005).

Findings from this study provided scientific validation of the efficacy of Falun Gong as a mind-body technique for health-wellness improvement (Q. Li et al., 2005), with plausible explanations for the remarkable healing benefits claimed by Falun Gong respondents in Falun Gong studies in mainland China (Author Unknown, 1998, 2002; Dan et al., 1998; Wang et al., 1998; Zhang & Xiao, 1996), Taiwan (Authors Unknown, 2003b; Lio et al., 2003), and North America (Authors Unknown, 1999, 2003a; Lowe, 2003; Ownby, 2003b, 2008a; S. J. Palmer, 2003; Porter, 2003). This was, however, a pilot study involving only a small sample size of six Falun Gong and six non–Falun Gong respondents. No other larger and similar studies have been conducted yet.

3.5 Non-research-based health-wellness Falun Gong literature

This subsection reviews some of the non-research-based Falun Gong literature focusing on health-wellness effects of Falun Gong. As indicated in Chapter 1, this dissertation intends to maintain reality and authenticity in the portrayal of Falun Gong and its health-wellness effects, ensuring the perceptions and experiences of both Falun Gong and non–Falun Gong respondents are conveyed respectfully.

Pullen (2000), a medical writer for Columbia Broadcasting System, presented a three-part health series on Falun Gong. She interviewed non–Falun Gong health professionals, an acupuncturist and a clinical psychologist, who acknowledged the healing potential of Falun Gong and its mind-body-spiritual approach (Pullen, 2000). Schechter (2000), journalist and author of *Falun Gong's Challenge to China*, also recognized the mind-body spiritual healing benefits of Falun Gong, and dedicated a chapter to "statements from practitioners around the world" (p. 128).

Gale and Gorman-Yao (2003) discussed the relevance and implications for nursing practice in providing culturally appropriate and sensitive nursing care to clients from diverse cultural and spiritual backgrounds. They believed

Falun Gong, with its "message of hope and spiritual renewal" (p. 125), and its beneficial effects such as physical and emotional health improvement, spiritual integrity, and the attainment of a high moral standard, could provide "solace and support" (p. 125) for both the individual and society in times of societal change (Gale & Gorman-Yao, 2003). Gale and Gorman-Yao (2003) recognized Falun Gong as the "most significant recent development in popular thinking about health and wellness in contemporary Chinese culture" (pp. 124-125).

Much has been written and published about the beneficial and trans-formational effects of Falun Gong by practitioners themselves. In the article, *Wellness - the better you*, a Canadian practitioner discussed how Falun Gong can offer a high-level wellness way of life across seven wellness domains, such as the physical, mental, emotional, social, spiritual, environmental, and occupational (Author Unknown, 2001). Personal accounts, often called "cultivation stories" (Clearwisdom editors, 2006, p. i), portray the insights of Falun Gong practitioners and their mind-body and spiritual healing journeys since starting Falun Gong practice. Collections of these stories have been published in books (Clearwisdom editors, 2006; Culp, n.d.; Life and hope renewed, 2005; McCoy & Zhang, n.d.), or as articles (Author Unknown, 2001; Galli, 2002; Yang, 2003; Yang & Nania, 2001) posted on Falun Gong websites, http://en.minghui.org and www.pureinsight.org, or presented at Falun Gong experience-sharing conferences around the world.

3.6 Effects of yoga on health

This section reviews literature exploring some of the effects of yoga. The word 'yoga' originates from Sanskrit (an ancient Indian language), literally meaning "union" (Oxford Dictionary, 2005, p. 1564). Yoga is defined as:

> *A Hindu spiritual and ascetic discipline, a part of which, including breath control, simple meditation, and the adoption of specific bodily postures, is widely practiced for health and relaxation (Oxford Dictionary, 2005, p. 2044).*

Yoga is described as a "mystic way of life" (p. 95), with a history of nearly 3000 years, from India (Singh, 2006). It is considered a mind-body practice, part of CAM (Atkinson & Permuth-Levine, 2009), and a "meditative movement" (C. E. Rogers et al., 2009, p. 246) practice. Yoga is generally regarded as a form of moderate physical exercise with three main aspects: postures (asanas); stretching and breathing techniques (pranayama); and meditation (dhyana) (Khalsa, 2003, 2004). There are diverse styles and different schools of yogic practices (Singh, 2006). Singh (2006) listed eight main styles of yoga, which includes hatha and raja yoga. Hatha yoga is the most widely popularized in Western society, while raja yoga comprises the highest form of yoga with the goal of "spiritual purification and self-understanding leading to Samadhi or union with the divine" (Oxford Dictionary, 2005, p. 2044).

Atkinson and Permuth-Levine (2009) noted the increasing use of yoga in the United States. It is widely used in adjunct to mainstream therapies for different conditions (Atkinson & Permuth-Levine, 2009; Carson et al., 2007; Khalsa, 2003; Singh, 2006; C. Smith, Hancock, Blake-Mortimer, & Eckert, 2007). In 2004, 7.5% of Americans practiced yoga at least once in their lifetime compared to 3.8% the year before (Atkinson & Permuth-Levine, 2009). Singh (2006) noted that hatha, mantra, and raja yoga were mainly used for psycho-emotional conditions, alluding to Patanjali's yoga sutras in the fourth century when yoga was used as therapy for psychosomatic disorders. The word "sutra" is of Sanskrit origin meaning rules, guidelines, or sacred writings (Oxford Dictionary, 2005).

Literature reviewed on yoga indicated that yoga-based interventions were shown to have beneficial effects for different health and medical conditions (Atkinson & Permuth-Levine, 2009; Author Unknown, 2009b; Carson et al., 2007; KueiMin Chen et al., 2009; Danhauer et al., 2009; Khalsa, 2003, 2004; Singh, 2006; C. Smith et al., 2007). Yoga was found to be beneficial for anxiety disorders, carpal tunnel syndrome, increased self-awareness and enhanced well-being, musculoskeletal problems, pain relief, and stress reduction (Girodo, 1974). Studies on yoga interventions covered different conditions, including the effects of yoga on women living with cancer (Carson et al., 2007; Danhauer et al., 2009; Galantino, 2003; Targ & Levine, 2002; Vadiraja et al., 2009), changes in heart rate, physical effects of yoga postures (Cowen & Adams, 2005, 2007), management of anxiety and stress reduction (Girodo, 1974; Javnbakhta, Kenari, & Ghasemi, 2009; C. Smith et al., 2007), regulation and perception of pain (Kakigi et al., 2005), mental health promotion and wellness maintenance for older adults (KueiMin Chen et al., 2009), and remediation for adolescent sex offenders (Derezotes, 2000).

Findings from the randomized comparative trial of yoga and relaxation by Smith, Hancock, Blake-Mortimer, and Eckert (2007) demonstrated that yoga was more effective than relaxation in enhancing mental health, just as effective as relaxation in reducing stress and anxiety, and for enhancing the general health status of respondents. Derezotes' (2000) study indicated an overall improvement in adolescents' ability to self-regulate and control their impulsive outbursts of anger and sexual aggression after a yoga intervention program. A Taiwan RCT study showed significant improvement in sleep quality, depression, and health status of older adults after commencing a yoga program specially tailored for their age (KueiMin Chen et al., 2009). Yoga has also been advocated as an adjunct therapy for women undergoing infertility treatment, experiencing the challenges of peri-menopause, and for menopause itself, although its efficacy remains unsubstantiated (Khalsa, 2003, 2004).

In a systematic review of RCT studies on meditation practices used in health care over the past 15 years, a total of 46 yoga studies were found involving healthy respondents, while 59 studies focused on clinical populations (Ospina et al., 2008). The RCTs on clinical populations included hypertension (8), asthma (7), heart ailments (7), type 2 diabetes (5), substance abuse (3), anxiety, chronic pain, and rheumatoid arthritis (2 each), and a multiple-factor study including cancer, epilepsy, multiple sclerosis, migraine and tension headaches, and pregnancy (Ospina et al., 2008, p. 1206). Overall, the methodological standard of the RCTs was not good and hence firm conclusions could not be drawn on efficacy (Ospina et al., 2008). Whilst RCTs are necessary, it may be justifiable to use a mixed quantitative and qualitative method approach to evaluate the effects of meditation (Ospina et al., 2008).

While most studies exploring the effects of yoga indicated positive benefits on various health and medical conditions, one RCT on yoga yielded no conclusive benefits or side effects of a yoga intervention on type 2 diabetes (Skoro-Kondza, Tai, Gadelrab, Drincevic, & Greenhalgh, 2009). Research problems, such as recruitment difficulties, respondents' ages, low motivation, and lack of compliance, meant a modified yoga program tailored to their specific needs was required (Skoro-Kondza et al., 2009). Researchers noted class, ethnicity, and age biases in yoga involvement, that yoga, like other CAM or mind-body therapies, seemed to attract younger, professional, and more educated white middle-class individuals (Skoro-Kondza et al., 2009). Other studies also indicated that the use of CAM, yoga, and mind-body therapies were closely linked with socio-demographic factors, such as age (Wu et al., 2007), ethnicity (Barnes et al., 2004; Wu et al., 2007), higher education level (Astin, 1998; Barnes et al., 2004; Mehta et al., 2007; Upchurch et al., 2007; Wu et al., 2007), income, and employment status (Upchurch et al., 2007; Wu et al., 2007). Women were more inclined to use mind-body therapies and to partake in yoga and other meditative movement practices (Barnes et al., 2004; Mehta et al., 2007; Upchurch et al., 2007).

Atkinson and Permuth-Levine (2009) explored the perceived benefits and barriers to yoga practice, finding that both the yoga and non-yoga participants perceived yoga as beneficial for mind-body health-wellness improvement. Their findings indicated that yoga has a health-wellness maintenance potential, and that health educators, counselors, and other health professionals can promote it as a "positive health behavior" (p. 12), or a health-wellness lifestyle choice for different individuals and communities (Atkinson & Permuth-Levine, 2009).

3.7 Effects of tai chi on health

This section provides a brief overview of literature exploring the effects of tai chi. Tai chi is a popular traditional Chinese form of exercise that integrates breathing techniques with rhythmic, continuous, dance-like meditative movements (Sandlund & Norlander, 2000). Tai chi is a form of "meditative movement" (C. E. Rogers et al., 2009, p. 246) practice. Like yoga and qigong, the National Center of Complementary and Alternative Medicine (NCCAM) has classified tai chi as part of CAM, a type of MBM, and described it as a "moving meditation" (NCCAM, 2009, p. 1). Zan Sanfeng, a 12th century Taoist monk, was believed to be the creator of tai chi as a self-defense form of martial art (NCCAM, 2009). Entrenched in Chinese Taoist philosophy, yin-yang theory and vital energy flow, tai chi is also considered a form of Chinese yoga (Sandlund & Norlander, 2000). It is a widely accepted form of gentle exercise regime especially for older adults in China, Asia, and other parts of the world (NCCAM, 2009). This slow, low-impact form of traditional Chinese exercise practiced to improve the quality of life of older people is gaining popularity in the United States as an adjunct to conventional treatment for age-related medical conditions (Author Unknown, 2009a; F. Li, McAuley, Harmer, Duncan, & Chaumeton, 2001; NCCAM, 2009). The NCCAM (2009) website describes the origin, key principles, health benefits, and also provides guidelines about tai chi and CAM use.

Tai chi offers many benefits for health-wellness maintenance of individuals who engage in it (Author Unknown, 2009a; NCCAM, 2009). Most of the studies reviewed focused on the effects of tai chi on older adults (Author Unknown, 2009a; Braithwaite, Griffin, Stephens, Murphy, & Marrow, 1998; Hogan, 2005; Irwin, Olmstead, & Oxman, 2007; Irwin, Pike, Cole, & Oxman, 2003; F. Li, Duncan et al., 2001; F. Li, McAuley et al., 2001; C. E. Rogers et al., 2009; Sandlund & Norlander, 2000; Sattin, Easley, Wolf, Chen, & Kutner, 2005; Voukelatos, Cumming, Lord, & Rissel, 2007; Yeh et al., 2004). Nearly 80% of studies from the PsychLit and Medline databases focused on the health-wellness effects of tai chi for the ageing population (Sandlund & Norlander, 2000).

Sandlund and Norlander (2000) evaluated studies on the effects of tai chi for stress reduction, health promotion, and wellness maintenance. Their review suggested tai chi may have positive benefits for older adults in the following areas: improved balance; reduced fear of falling; higher oxygen uptake; greater flexibility; muscle relaxation; enhanced lateral body stability; reduced anxiety; lower percentage of body fat; and normalized blood pressure (Sandlund & Norlander, 2000, p. 145). The length of time respondents engaged in tai chi practice was influential in gauging its potential therapeutic health-wellness benefits (Sandlund & Norlander, 2000). Sandlund and Norlander (2000) identified three omissions in their review: studies on the effects of tai chi on younger and middle-aged respondents; gender aspects; and an absence of comparison with other similar meditative movement practices.

Hogan's work (2005) specifically reviewed the effects of tai chi for older adults and identified that this form of meditative movement practice could have health-wellness benefits for the ageing population. The benefits included physical resilience with better balance, fewer falls, improved cardiovascular, respiratory, postural, and musculoskeletal functioning, and cognitive resilience as in enhanced mood, positive emotions, and maintenance of the central nervous system functioning (Hogan, 2005). F. Li et al. (2001) also found tai chi to be beneficial for health-wellness maintenance for older adults through improved self-efficacy and positive changes in exercise behavior. An Australian RCT examining the effects of tai chi in preventing falls in older adults demonstrated that tai chi could reduce falls (Voukelatos et al., 2007). Given the potential benefits and low cost as an intervention program, tai chi can improve quality of life, boost resilience, and may have health care and medical cost-saving benefits for the ageing population (Hogan, 2005; F. Li, McAuley et al., 2001).

A recent systematic review of RCTs on meditation practices used in health care identified 25 studies on tai chi with healthy respondents and 21 focusing on medical conditions (Ospina et al., 2008). RCTs on clinical populations included a variety of medical conditions ranging from cancer, depression, osteoarthritis, stroke, and cardiovascular illness (Ospina et al., 2008, pp. 1205-1206). Ospina et al. (2008) noted the poor quality of the methodological standard of most of the RCTs and stated that it might be justifiable to use a mixed methods approach to evaluate the effects of meditative movement practices.

Findings from a recent review of 36 RCTs involving nearly 3,800 respondents suggested that both tai chi and qigong practices have definite benefits for older adults (C. E. Rogers et al., 2009). However, spirituality and the reference to the positive link between spirituality and health are absent from these studies, despite it being a vital aspect of these Eastern meditative practices and playing a vital role in healthy and positive ageing (C. E. Rogers et al., 2009).

Voukelatos et al's (2007) RCT triggered a response that "any intervention may have provided the same beneficial results" (p. 776), and also the question of whether the findings of reduced falls in elderly respondents were due to tai chi, placebo, or Hawthorne effect (Katz, 2008). The researchers responded stating their results were consistent with other studies, suggesting an inverse Hawthorne effect in a more recent study, which indicated an increase in falls (Cumming, Voukelatos, Lord, & Rissel, 2008). Placebo effect refers to a beneficial effect or "clinically significant response to a therapeutically inert substance or non-specific treatment," (VandenBos, 2007, p. 705). Hawthorne effect is defined as "the effect on the behavior of individuals of knowing that they are being observed or are taking part in research" (VandenBos, 2007, p. 430), hence producing a beneficial effect and a better than normal result

(McCarney et al., 2007). It originated from the name of the suburb of the Western Electric Company where the occurrence was first observed in the 1920s in a series of studies on productivity (M. Chiesa & Hobbs, 2008; Hindle, 2008; McCarney et al., 2007; Oxford Dictionary, 2005; VandenBos, 2007).

Katz's (2008) reference to Hawthorne effect in the tai chi RCT raised a valid point for researchers confronted by critics and writers who used Hawthorne effect, halo effect (Oh & Ramaprasad, 2003; Thorndike, 1920), and social desirability effect (Booth-Kewley, Larson, & Miyoshi, 2007; Kuentzel, Henderson, & Melville, 2008; VandenBos, 2007) to dispute or discredit research findings as biased, erroneous, and under the influence of these phenomena. Halo effect is defined as a "marked tendency to think of the person in general as rather good or rather inferior and to color the judgments of the qualities by this general feeling" (Oh & Ramaprasad, 2003, p. 319; Thorndike, 1920, p. 25), that is, letting a general impression influence evaluation of other specific aspects. Social desirability effect refers to "a bias that prompts individuals to present themselves in ways that are likely to be seen as positive" (VandenBos, 2007, p. 864). It refers to respondents' tendency to over-report in self-report surveys to make themselves look good or to create a positive impression (Booth-Kewley et al., 2007; Silverthorn & Gekoski, 1995).

Chiesa and Hobbs (2008), in their critical review on the usefulness of Hawthorne effect in social research, presented several different and contradictory definitions of Hawthorne effect in textbooks and journal articles, and provided their rationale against its usage:

> Given its multiple, contradictory, and imprecise meanings, the HE cannot be used effectively to prompt an examination of what alternative events may have influenced experimental findings. Challenged to consider the possibility of a Hawthorne Effect in a journal submission or conference presentation, how is an author or presenter to know which of the multiple meanings a questioner is alluding? Is the questioner referring to the presence of others, or to the warmth of the climate, or to expectations, attitudes or beliefs? Or is the term used to refer to awareness or unconscious effects? Perhaps a particular questioner is referring to an uncontrolled effect of special attention, artificial conditions, novelty, innovation, change or variety.

Without specification of which or what type of uncontrolled-for variable is referred to, an author or a presenter is at a loss to defend their research against the challenge of a possible Hawthorne Effect.

Where concerns about research methods or experimental control arise, critics have a responsibility to specify their concerns more precisely. It is also inappropriate for authors to employ the term in interpreting their own results since, given its multiple meanings, it provides no useful information for readers in terms of evaluating specific controlling effects (M. Chiesa & Hobbs, 2008, p. 73).

Nonetheless, Hawthorne effect, halo, and social desirability effects often crop up in research, and hence deserve the researcher's attention, understanding, and awareness of their existence and the possibility of such occurrences.

3.8 Effects of qigong on health

This section provides a brief overview of studies exploring the effects of qigong. Qigong has been described as an ancient Chinese self-healing art, technique or health practice (Kevin Chen, 2000; Leung & Singhal, 2004; M. Li, Chen, & Mo, 2002; Sancier, 1999). Tai chi is also considered a type of qigong (Author Unknown, 2009a; C. E. Rogers et al., 2009; Sancier, 1999). Qigong is defined as "a Chinese system of exercises and breathing control related to tai chi" (Oxford Dictionary, 2005, p. 1436).

There are different schools and styles of qigong developed by different qigong masters for health-wellness maintenance (C. E. Rogers et al., 2009). Qigong, in its simplest explanation, is a generic term referring to different schools and styles of a traditional Chinese form of energy exercises and meditative movement practices. As discussed in Chapter One, Falun Gong was first introduced to the public as a form of qigong in 1992 (Ownby, 2008a; D. Palmer, 2007; Parker, 2004; Penny, 2001; Porter, 2003). Mr. Li Hongzhi, the founder of Falun Gong, explained that qigong is an ancient Chinese cultivation practice with a "newly crafted term that complies with modern people's mindset" (H. Li, 2001b, p. 27). The word qigong was first coined in the early 1950s (Xu, 1999). Escalating interest in qigong as a practice for health and wellness maintenance began in the 1980s in mainland China when many qigong masters began to teach a variety of qigong in public (Ownby, 2008a; D. Palmer, 2007; Xu, 1999).

Like other meditative movement practices, such as yoga and tai chi, qigong was reported to have beneficial effects and health-wellness maintenance potential (Leung & Singhal, 2004; C. E. Rogers et al., 2009; Sancier, 1996, 1999). There were numerous studies conducted in mainland China exploring the effects of qigong, but not many were empirical (Sancier, 1999). Few Chinese studies on qigong were published because of translation problems, limited study details, and few suitable journals to publish findings (Sancier, 1996). It could also be argued that many qigong studies conducted in mainland China failed to meet the Western scientific standards (Ai, 2003). Ai (2003) reasoned that the study limitations could be attributed to the conflict of applying a Western scientific and clinical model of research to qigong, which is a holistic, Eastern meditative movement and spiritual practice based on the philosophy of the intangible vital flow of energy, that is beyond the realm of science. She proposed applying the wellness model to future studies for a more holistic evaluation instead of the clinical and illness approach (Ai, 2003).

Sancier (1996; 1999) reviewed studies exploring qigong use in medical settings and effects of qigong with medication for medical conditions such as asthma, cancer, and hypertension. His review suggested that the integration of qigong and pharmacology may have beneficial effects such as lower dosage, fewer instances of stroke and mortality, less sick leave, and reduced hospitalization and medical costs (Sancier, 1999). Reduction in individual and public health and medical costs would be an attractive benefit of qigong and other meditative movement practices (F. Li, McAuley et al., 2001; Sancier & Holman, 2004).

Two RCTs investigating effects of Korean qigong indicated its benefits in alleviating the symptoms of premenstrual syndrome (Jang & Lee, 2004; Jang, Lee, Kim, & Chong, 2004), and evidence-based studies on Korean qigong demonstrated positive effects for heart rate variations (M. S. Lee et al., 2002), neuroendocrine, and immune functions (M. S. Lee, Jeong, Jang, Ryu, & Moon, 2003; M. S. Lee, Kang, Ryu, & Moon, 2004; M. S. Lee & Ryu, 2004) and blood-gas concentrations (M. S. Lee, Ryu, Song, & Moon, 2004). A case study on two cancer patients also found beneficial effects of Korean qigong, such as alleviation of anxiety, pain and discomfort (M. S. Lee & Jang, 2005).

Ospina et al. (2008) found two qigong studies on healthy respondents and 11 on clinical populations. The clinical RCTs included hypertension and a variety of medical conditions, including fibromyalgia, muscular dystrophy, diabetes, and substance abuse (Ospina et al., 2008, p. 1205). Sound methodological quality was found lacking from most of the RCTs, highlighting the need for more research rigor to achieve greater reliability and validity, and the use of a mixed methods approach to evaluate the effects of qigong and other meditative movement practices (Ospina et al., 2008).

An RCT examining the effects of qigong found significant reduction in anxiety and qigong's potential to elicit positive psychological effects (Johansson, Hassmen, & Jouper, 2008). The researchers proposed health professionals should recommend qigong for its mental health benefits and for health-wellness promotion (Johansson et al., 2008). Another RCT demonstrating the use of the eight section brocades qigong as an alternative psychosocial intervention in geriatric rehabilitative care indicated qigong's potential as an alternative health-wellness program for older individuals with chronic physical ailments (Tsang, Mok, Au-Yeung, & Chan, 2003).

Given its potential benefits and the low cost of these programs, qigong (like other meditative movement practices) may have public health and medical cost benefits for the ageing population. A recent review of RCTs on the effects of qigong for older adults found more significant physical health improvement and less conclusive psychological effects on depression (C. E. Rogers et al., 2009). The element of spirituality and the link between spirituality/health, which is a vital aspect of these Eastern meditative movement practices, was again absent from these studies (C. E. Rogers et al., 2009).

3.9 The link between spirituality/religion and health

Eastern meditation disciplines and meditative movement practices have a strong spiritual component (C. E. Rogers et al., 2009). It is therefore relevant to review literature exploring the link between spirituality/religion and health, as it provides the theoretical framework for this dissertation. Numerous Australian and U.S. empirical studies have indicated a positive link between spirituality/ religion and health, with an increasing body of evidence demonstrating that spirituality/religion plays a vital role in the health and well-being of the individual, and in their medical care (Coruh et al., 2005; Haynes et al., 2007; Hilbers et al., 2007; Koenig, 1999, 2004a, 2004b, 2007; Koenig & Cohen, 2002; Koenig et al., 2001; Maselko & Kubzansky, 2006; Peach, 2003; Williams & Sternthal, 2007).

Findings from an Australian study conducted at the Prince of Wales Hospital (POWH) in Sydney demonstrated that:

- Spirituality/religion is important to 74% of POWH patients;
- More than 80% of patients reported spiritual/religious beliefs influence health and become more significant during illness;
- 80% reported rituals and spiritual/religious practices offer self-care support, therapy, comfort, meaning, and connection during their illness;
- Spirituality/religion plays a vital role in health care decision-making; and
- Spirituality/religion can be a resource, coping strategy, or a psychosocial support mechanism for patients (Haynes et al., 2007, p. 1; Hilbers et al., 2007, pp. 27-28).

These findings were consistent with other studies showing a positive link between spirituality/religion and health (Koenig, 2004a; Koenig et al., 2001; Williams & Sternthal, 2007). Koenig (2004a; 2004b; 2001) summarized studies (nearly 2,000 by 2002) examining the relationship between spirituality/ religion and better physical and mental health, enhanced wellness, and better quality of life. He explained how spirituality/religion offers "comfort, hope and meaning, particularly in coping with a medical illness" (Koenig, 2004a, p. 1195). Koenig (2004a; 2004b) confirmed that spiritual and religious beliefs and practices are linked with:

- Less anxiety;
- Less substance abuse;
- Less depression and quicker recovery;
- Lower suicide rates;
- Enhanced well-being, higher sense of hope and optimism;
- More purpose and meaning in life;
- Increased social support;

- Greater marital satisfaction and stability (2004a, p. 1195);
- A more positive world view;
- Better psychological coping and integration of traumatic life events;
- A sense of control and personal empowerment; and
- Positive role models to foster endurance and acceptance of situations that cannot be changed (Koenig, 2004a, p. 1195, 2004b, p. 78).

In *The link between religion and health: Psychoneuroimmunology and the faith factor* (Koenig & Cohen, 2002), Koenig (2002) presented a chapter exploring the connection between psychoneuroimmunology (PNI) and religion. Spiritual/religious beliefs, rituals and practices were shown to foster positive and healthy behaviors, such as lower alcohol consumption and cigarette smoking, and discourage unhealthy behaviors like substance use, risky sexual practices, and other unsafe activities (Koenig & Cohen, 2002). Nearly 80% of studies exploring this link reported a positive relationship between spirituality/religion and health (Koenig & Cohen, 2002; Koenig et al., 2001). Numerous studies also indicated the positive link between spirituality/ religion and health, and demonstrated how spirituality/religion contributed to better health, positive emotions, wellness, life satisfaction, and feelings of contentment in individuals (Coruh et al., 2005; Haynes et al., 2007; Hilbers et al., 2007; Koenig, 1999, 2004a, 2004b, 2007; Koenig & Cohen, 2002; Koenig et al., 2001; Maselko & Kubzansky, 2006; Peach, 2003; Rippentrop et al., 2005; Weaver et al., 2003; Williams & Sternthal, 2007; Yeager et al., 2006).

Being happy and cultivating positive emotions, such as optimism, joy, happiness, contentment, and serenity, can optimize health and wellness (Fredrickson, 2000; Lemonick, 2005; Wallis, 2005). Relaxation techniques, yoga, and meditative practices that elicit the "Relaxation Response" (Crombie, 2002; G. D. Jacobs, 2001), tranquility, contentment, and other positive emotions, can buffer against negative emotions and hence promote better health and wellness (Fredrickson, 2000). Koenig (2004b) provided an explanation for this:

> By enhancing positive emotions such as well-being, hope, and a sense of
> purpose and meaning in life, religious beliefs and practices may help to
> counteract the negative stressors that set off the fight-flight response. The
> flight-fight response, when allowed to proceed unimpeded, produces changes

in immune function, cortisol and epinephrine levels, blood pressure, and
cardiac function that interfere with health and healing (Koenig, 2004b, p. 80).

Besides hope, sense of purpose, and meaning in life, other reasons for the positive link between spirituality/religion and better health include a sense of self-control, positive role models of biblical and spiritual leaders, and social support from the spiritual/religious community (Koenig, 2004b). Weaver et al. (2003) noted that spiritual/religious practices can support coping during crises and traumatic experiences. Rippentrop et al. (2005) examined the link between spirituality/religion and health and chronic pain, finding cost savings and health benefits for individuals with chronic pain. They advised that no causal relationship could be drawn from their cross-sectional study (Rippentrop et al., 2005).

Williams and Sternthal (2007) provided an overview of Australian and U.S. studies on spirituality/religion and health, and reported a positive link between spiritual/religious involvement and healthy behaviors , implying that this could have a lifestyle balancing effect. There is strong empirical evidence of a positive link between religious attendance/participation and longer life expectancy, that is, higher religious involvement is linked with lower mortality risk (Williams & Sternthal, 2007).

Williams & Sternthal (2007) also discussed the potential negative effects of religion on health, such as religious guilt, expectations and fears, over-dependence on faith healing, and negative religious coping. Rippentrop et al. (2005) found negative effects as well. Thus, while spirituality/religion plays a vital and positive role in health and wellness and better quality of life, certain religious beliefs and spiritual conflicts may hinder and interfere with patient care and medical treatment (Koenig, 2004a, 2004b). These negative effects included "excessive guilt, obsessive preoccupations, worries, or social ostracism" (Koenig, 2004b, p. 79), religious beliefs against using antibiotics, having immunizations, and accepting blood or medical treatment (Koenig, 2004a).

Researchers not only identified conflicts from patients, but also from health professionals for not addressing spirituality/religion in health care practice due to various reasons, such as lack of time, discomfort and uncertainty arising from lack of knowledge, training, experience, and fear of overstepping their area of expertise (Haynes et al., 2007; Hilbers et al., 2007; Koenig, 2004a). Hilbers et al. (2007) observed that the spirituality/religion and health link can be negative, neutral or positive. However, findings from their POWH Sydney study did indicate a strong positive link (Haynes et al., 2007; Hilbers et al., 2007). Koenig (2004b) noted that there were too few RCTs to establish causal links between spirituality/religion and health. Future studies should investigate causal effects of spirituality/religion on better health-wellness to determine definitive conclusions. While numerous studies have demonstrated a positive link between spirituality/religion and health, this relationship demands ongoing attention, with more rigorous RCTs and also the use of the mixed methods approach to study their effects on health and wellness.

3.10 Summary

This concludes Chapter 3, which has introduced the aim, objective, scope of studies investigating the health-wellness effects of Falun Gong, and an extensive literature review. Lack of studies investigating the health-wellness effects of Falun Gong rendered it necessary not only to review existing literature on Falun Gong, but also to examine the health-wellness effects of other similar Eastern meditation practices, including, yoga, tai chi, and qigong, to provide a sound rationale for embarking on this health-wellness research on Falun Gong. This review comprised different aspects of meditation, historical contexts, trends in meditative/spiritual practices, the role of meditation in the helping professions, effects of meditation, other meditative movement practices, and existing Falun Gong literature.

The link between spirituality/religion and health, which forms the theoretical framework of this research, has also been reviewed. There are numerous studies on meditation, yoga, tai chi and qigong that demonstrated their beneficial health-wellness effects. In the attempt to broaden the scope of the literature review, these different Eastern meditative movement practices were included, but to a limited extent, to avoid verbosity.

Findings from the literature reviewed indicated consistent beneficial effects of meditation, Falun Gong, and other meditative movement practices, and their potential to promote health and maintain wellness. This review has also established the positive link between spirituality/religion and health, and its vital role in health-wellness maintenance. It has achieved its aim and objective, and offered greater insight into the dynamics and the health-wellness effects of Falun Gong and other mind-body meditative movement practices. Finally, the review has provided a solid rationale and highlighted the need to carry out this research in investigating the health-wellness potential of Falun Gong. Chapter 4 will present the design for this research.

CHAPTER 4

Research Design

4.1 Chapter overview

This chapter discusses the research design, approach, and methods used for this research. This research was designed as a descriptive cross-sectional online survey using a mixed methods approach of mainly quantitative data with some qualitative data collection. The research comprised two parts: Part A was to obtain a global demographic profile of Falun Gong (Falun Dafa) practitioners, including age group, ethnicity, country of birth and residence, education level, occupation, and gross annual household income. Part B, the primary component of the research, was to investigate the health-wellness effects of Falun Gong as perceived by individuals who practice Falun Gong. This research seeks to ascertain any observed differences or similarities between Falun Gong and non–Falun Gong individuals in terms of their demographic profile and health-wellness statuses, and whether individuals who practice Falun Gong experience better health and wellness than those who do not.

This chapter describes the three different phases of the research: Development phase; data collection phase; and data processing phase. It also provides a rationale for the choice of the research design, the use of self-reporting, the self-designed survey questions and the Short Form (SF-36) Health Survey (Brazier et al., 1992; Garratt, Ruta, Abdalla, Buckingham, & Russell, 1993; Jenkinson, Coulter, & Wright, 1993; McHorney, Ware, Lu, & Sherbourne, 1994; Ware Jr., 2008; Ware Jr. & Sherbourne, 1992).

4.2 Research design

This section will discuss the design, approach, and method adopted for this research, as well as the rationale for the choice of research design.

4.2.1 Study design and approach

This Falun Gong research adopted a mixed methods approach, which is frequently used in counseling psychology and social sciences research (Hanson, Creswell, Clark, Petska, & Creswell, 2005; Miles & Huberman, 1994; Sandelowski, 2000). The mixed methods approach was used to broaden the scope, provide deeper insights, and enhance the analytical strength of the research (Hanson et al., 2005; Miles & Huberman, 1994; Sandelowski, 2000). The data collection process involved concurrent implementation of the mixed quantitative and qualitative approach in a single anonymous online survey. The online survey was chosen because of its convenience in administration to a large sample of respondents from around the world. The quantitative method was prioritized and emphasized because it was an effective way to collect data, while the qualitative items aimed to enhance the quality of this research and provide more insights into the findings.

Two anonymous online surveys were conducted: the Health and Wellness Survey One (HW1) for Falun Gong respondents; and the Health and Wellness Survey Two (HW2) for non–Falun Gong respondents. Both surveys were administered via the Internet using the University of South Australia TellUs2 online survey tool. The two online surveys consisted of items with a range of options for respondents to choose, including several with text box options for written responses up to 2000 characters. Both the quantitative and qualitative data comprised self-reports from the self-designed questionnaire (to be explained further in this chapter) and the SF-36 Health Survey (Brazier et al., 1992; Garratt et al., 1993; Jenkinson et al., 1993; McHorney et al., 1994; Ware Jr., 2008; Ware Jr. & Sherbourne, 1992).

4.2.2 Methods

A descriptive, cross-sectional survey enabled comparison between two groups of respondents. The aim was to describe and explain the demographic and health-wellness characteristics of two groups of respondents. Their age group, gender, ethnicity, relationship status, education level, occupation, including other demographic details, and the self-reports of their health and wellness have been captured at a particular point in time during the specified data collection period. Descriptive studies describe *what is,* while surveys examine a specific group or groups of respondents (Hadley & Mitchell, 1995; Heppner, Kivlighan, & Wampold, 1999) and cross-sectional studies collect data at one particular point in time to provide a snapshot of the characteristics of the specified group (Spector, 1994). The survey method is one of the most frequently used research methods in social sciences and counseling research because it is a simple, inexpensive method of data collection and easy to administer to a large sample of respondents (Heppner et al., 1999). It is also convenient and easy to administer via the Internet. The self-administered Internet survey method was used in this research because of its benefits, which included ease, convenience of administration, and elimination of data entry costs and errors (Booth-Kewley et al., 2007). It was also used as a precautionary measure to maintain "social distance" (Heerwegh, 2009, p. 112) and to reduce or eliminate the influence of social desirability effects (Heerwegh, 2009; Tourangeau, Couper, & Steiger, 2003; VandenBos, 2007).

An anonymous online survey method was chosen for this research because it was deemed the most effective way to reach out to Falun Gong respondents globally. It has been documented that Falun Gong is practiced in over 100 countries around the world (Falun Dafa Association, 2009b). A visit to the Falun Gong website, (www.falundafa.org), gives a clear indication of the worldwide Falun Gong network. Existing Falun Gong studies used the Internet survey method (Lowe, 2003) and provided a good insight into the important role of the Internet for Falun Gong practitioners (Porter, 2003). Emails, meetings, and Falun Gong websites are important communication tools for Falun Gong practitioners because the Internet offers a fast and inexpensive way to keep abreast with Falun Gong-related news and online articles, and to communicate with other practitioners from different regions and around the world (Porter, 2003).

One of the limitations of cross-sectional studies is that causal inferences are not possible (Spector, 1994) and hence no causal conclusions can be drawn from cross-sectional studies. Hadley and Mitchell (1995) clarified that the purpose of a purely descriptive study was not to establish causality. Neither is it the aim of this research. Despite the limitations of the descriptive cross-sectional study, this method is useful in providing a snapshot of the demographic and health-wellness profile of Falun Gong and non–Falun Gong respondents.

4.2.3 Self-reporting

Self-reporting forms the basis of survey studies (Northrup, 1996; Spector, 1994) and is often used in social sciences and counseling research (Barker, Pistrang, & Elliot, 2005; Heppner et al., 1999). Survey studies often rely on self-reports to obtain demographic data and individual characteristics including attitudes, behaviors, values, or beliefs of respondents (Heppner et al., 1999). Self-reporting involves having respondents assess and report the answers themselves on the basis that they will answer the items spontaneously and honestly.

There are benefits and limitations to using self-reporting (Barker et al., 2005; Donaldson & Grant-Vallone, 2002; Heppner et al., 1999; Prince et al., 2008; Razavi, 2001; Spector, 1994). The rationale for its use in this descriptive survey includes numerous benefits:

- Convenient to use as an online survey;
- Practical, time-efficient, low cost, and inexpensive to administer;
- Simplicity and ease in self-administration to a large sample;
- Obtaining respondents' own perspectives and perceptions;
- No specific skills required from the researcher or respondents;
- Respondents can complete survey privately and in their own time; and
- Respondents' confidentiality is ensured (Barker et al., 2005; Heppner et al., 1999; Prince et al., 2008).

Self-report methods are not without their limitations. One of the main criticisms concerns the validity and reliability of data due to the subjective nature of the respondents' responses to surveys (Barker et al., 2005; Donaldson & Grant-Vallone, 2002; Heppner et al., 1999; Prince et al., 2008; Razavi, 2001; Spector, 1994). Other limitations include:

- Respondents not always being honest and truthful;
- Misreporting either from under or over-reporting; and

- Distortions of the truth, either deliberately or unconsciously, to create a positive or a better impression (Barker et al., 2005; Donaldson & Grant-Vallone, 2002; Heppner et al., 1999; Prince et al., 2008; Razavi, 2001; Spector, 1994).

This tendency for respondents to give answers to create a good impression, known as the social desirability effect (VandenBos, 2007), has been recognized as a limitation of self-report studies (Booth-Kewley et al., 2007; Kuentzel et al., 2008). Despite its limitations, the self-report survey could offer worthwhile information and should not be rejected as a mediocre methodology (Spector, 1994). Spector (1994) advised that the self-report survey should be used for what it is designed to do. Northrup (1996) rationalized that self-report surveys are designed to elicit honesty, that respondents are more likely to tell the truth since participation in most self-report surveys is voluntary and the researcher often stresses the importance of the respondents' views and their contribution.

Self-reporting is highly relevant and valuable in counseling research (Barker et al., 2005; Heppner et al., 1999). In designing this research, the researcher adopted Carl Rogers' person-centered "the client knows best" (Mearns & Thorne, 2007, p. 1) stance that respondents know best how to self-assess their general health-wellness status. Since clients' thoughts and feelings are the central focus in therapeutic interactions (Heppner et al., 1999), in the same way the respondents' perceptions of their own health-wellness status are important, relevant, and valuable to the researcher. The self-report survey can help to enhance our understanding of the real world of attitudes, behaviors, beliefs, and health-wellness status of the respondents. On balancing of the benefits and limitations, the self-report method was used to good effect.

4.2.4 Research process

This section discusses the research process, which comprises three phases: Development phase; data collection phase; and data processing phase. The data processing phase includes reporting, analysis, interpretation, and presentation of the findings. A flow chart was designed to illustrate the entire research process, as shown in Chart 4.1.

4.3 Development phase

This is the first phase, which included framing the research question, selecting the research methodology and design, identifying potential respondents, preparing the research information sheet (RIS) for respondents, designing survey questions, and establishing an international pilot study to obtain feedback on the self-designed questionnaire for HW1 and HW2. It involved commencing the literature review and applying for ethics approval with the University of South Australia's Human Research Ethics Committee (HREC) to conduct this research. The chairperson of the European Falun Dafa Association and the presidents of the three Australian Falun Dafa associations (New South Wales, Queensland, and Victoria Falun Dafa associations) were contacted at this time. As part of the ethics approval process, a letter was sent to the chairperson or presidents of the Australian and overseas Falun Dafa associations requesting help and cooperation to disseminate the RIS and seeking written approval to place the two online surveys on the Falun Gong websites.

Chart 4.1 Falun Gong health and wellness research flow chart

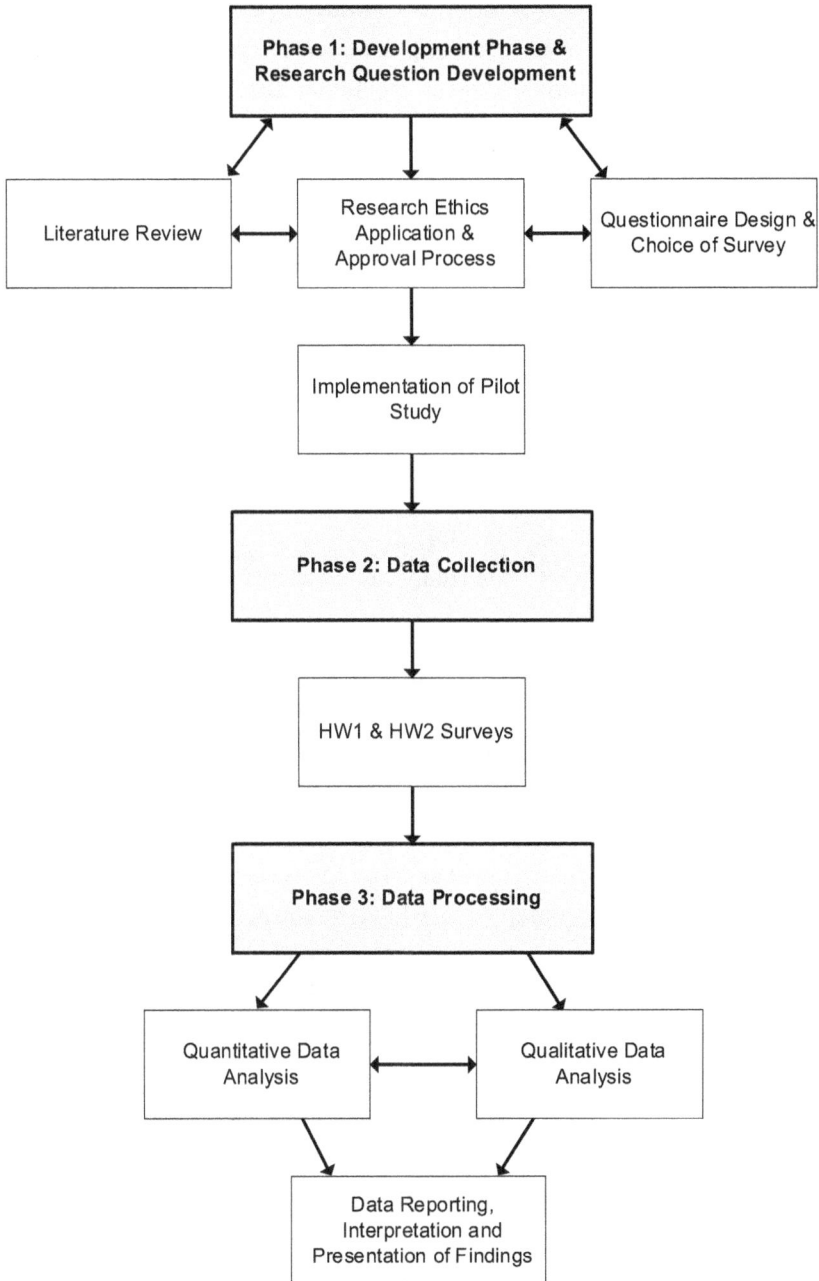

4.3.1 Research ethics protocol and approval process

The application for ethics approval was submitted to HREC on September 25, 2006. The HREC responded requesting the researcher to resubmit the ethics protocol (P21/06) and provided seven recommendations:

- Rephrase research question;
- Clarify how factors other than benefits of Falun Gong are not the cause for the health-wellness improvement of Falun Gong respondents;
- Suggestions for the self-designed questionnaire;
- Clarify how the researcher will prevent mainland Chinese Falun Gong (including Hong Kong) practitioners or those coming from mainland China from participating in the survey, given the Chinese Communist Party's (CCP) persecution of Falun Gong;
- Request Falun Dafa associations to place the URL web links of the HW1 and HW2 Surveys on the Falun Gong websites;
- Five suggestions for the RIS; and
- Obtain written approval from Falun Dafa associations before commencing research.

The ethics protocol (P21/06) was resubmitted on November 2, 2006, with changes based on the HREC's recommendations, which included the following:

- Provided rationale for demographic data collection;
- Amended self-designed questionnaire and the RIS;
- Explained that this research was based on the perceptions and self-reports from two groups of respondents, which can only be indicative and not to form any definitive causal conclusions from the findings;
- Obtained written letters of approval from different Falun Dafa associations and also permission to place web links of the online surveys on Falun Gong websites;
- Contacted the university information technology security specialist about Internet security and risk management;
- Inserted these two sentences in the RIS and the surveys: "The researcher will not be approaching Falun Gong practitioners in China to participate in the survey. Please do not complete the online survey if Falun Gong is banned in your country, or if participating poses a security risk for you and your family;" and

- Included the following paragraph in the RIS as requested by HREC: "The researcher will take every care to remove responses from any identifying material as early as possible. Likewise, individual responses will be kept confidential by the researcher and not be identified in the reporting of the research. However, researchers cannot guarantee the confidentiality or anonymity of material transferred by email or the Internet."

The HREC reviewed and approved the resubmission. Dr. John Court, principal supervisor at the time, and Associate Professor Heather Mattner of Southern Cross University, New South Wales, (principal supervisor upon Dr. John Court's retirement), supervised the ethics approval application, and the research process to ensure that it adhered to the ethics procedures and conditions stipulated in the ethics protocol. This research was thus conducted in accordance with the guidelines and rigors of the university's ethics protocol.

Care was undertaken to ensure that the research procedure not only adhered to the HREC's standards, but also the *National Statement on Ethical Conduct in Human Research* as stipulated by the National Health and Medical Research Council (NHMRC) to maintain research merit and integrity, justice, beneficence, and respect for research participants (NHMRC, 2007, pp. 12-13). This is because all human communications, including those in human research, carry ethical implications (NHMRC, 2007).

4.3.2 Research information for respondents

The research information developed comprised the Letter to Participants and the RIS (see Appendices 1 and 2 respectively). The one-page letter to respondents explained the purpose of the research, requesting potential Falun Gong respondents to complete HW1 and to invite their non–Falun Gong family members, friends, or colleagues to complete HW2.

The RIS was a two-page document with details about the research. It described the purpose, value of the research, and offered an overview of the research process, participation criteria, and instructions for potential respondents. The website URLs for HW1 and HW2 were provided in the RIS. The letter to respondents and the RIS were posted on Falun Gong websites and also emailed to pilot study members, key contact persons, and coordinators of other Falun Gong projects for dissemination to all potential respondents around the world.

4.4 The pilot study

The pilot study played a vital role in the research process. The main aim of the pilot study was to obtain feedback and recommendations from the panel before the actual online survey commenced. The secondary purpose was to inform pilot study members of the research process so that they could play a key role in helping to disseminate the research information to potential Falun Gong respondents. The pilot study objectives were:

1. To fulfill the initial stage of the research process proposed in the research ethics protocol;
2. To form a 'think tank' of individuals from different professional and education backgrounds to scrutinize the RIS and the questionnaire; and
3. To familiarize pilot study members with this research.

Chairperson/presidents of Falun Dafa associations and key Falun Dafa contact persons were selected as pilot study members. They provided a vital communication link between the researcher and Falun Gong respondents, and facilitated a 'research assistant' role to answer questions and explain the research procedures to potential respondents at Falun Gong activities and meetings across the world. During the data collection phase, the researcher took the precaution to contact only the pilot study members to minimize contact and keep a 'social distance' from potential respondents to avoid introducing response bias and reduce the influence of social desirability effect (VandenBos, 2007).

4.4.1 What the pilot study process entailed

The pilot study package comprised four items: 1) letter to respondents; 2) RIS; 3) self-designed questionnaires for HW1 and HW2; and 4) feedback sheet for pilot study members to complete and return to the researcher. The SF-36 Health Survey was excluded from the pilot study because it is a widely used, reliable, and well-validated general health assessment tool (Garratt et al., 1993; Jenkinson et al., 1993; Stanfeld, Roberts, & Foot, 1997; Ware Jr.,

2008). Its use has been authenticated in about 4,000 publications (Ware Jr., 2000, 2008).

Selection criteria for pilot study members were as follows:
- Chairperson or members of Falun Dafa associations or key contact persons;
- Education and professional knowledge of research;
- Recommendation from other pilot study team members; and
- Experienced Falun Gong practitioners.

One US member was invited due to a previous involvement in a Falun Gong wellness assessment conducted by the researcher in 2003. Non–Falun Gong individuals were excluded from the pilot study to keep it simple and straightforward. Falun Gong practitioners were the research target group. The pilot study commenced in May 2007. Pilot study members were from Australia, the United States, and the United Kingdom (U.K.). Communication between the researcher and the pilot study members was either by telephone or email. The pilot study package was emailed to ten participants. Reminders to return the completed feedback form were sent later. It took approximately two weeks for the completed feedback forms to be returned. The response rate was 90% (n=9). Several pilot study members provided extensive feedback. These comments and recommendations were discussed with the research supervisors at that time, Dr. J. Court and Dr. H. Mattner. The supervisors approved the recommendations upon ensuring that they would not affect the already approved research ethics protocol or violate HREC's conditions, and changes were accordingly made to the questionnaires and the RIS.

4.4.2 Pilot study feedback – summary

Feedback and recommendations from the pilot study team was useful and mostly pertained to rephrasing the self-designed survey questions. One participant noticed "Falun Dafa was not mentioned anywhere at all" in the RIS and commented that since the global survey included Falun Gong and non–Falun Gong respondents, it was not known whether Falun Gong would be more popularly known as Falun Dafa in certain countries. An explanation was added to the RIS stating, "Falun Gong is also known as Falun Dafa. For consistency, Falun Gong is used in all research materials."

Another comment related to the self-designed questions in HW2 for non–Falun Gong respondents, which asked them to rate their perceptions of Falun Gong respondents' health-wellness status instead of their own. Since reporting on the other was inconsistent with the self-reporting method used in this research, these questions were subsequently removed from HW2. It was also recommended that the term "meditation" be removed from the phrase "Falun Gong meditation" in the research title, as it might be confusing and misleading to potential Falun Gong and non–Falun Gong respondents.

Other changes following the pilot study process included:
- Adding questions on frequency and time spent on Falun Gong exercise practice and study of the teachings of Falun Gong;
- Revising the ethnicity question in Section One of HW1 and HW2;
- Inserting a statement to explain the term "first language;" and
- Rewording sentences in the RIS to reflect greater clarity and accuracy.

One pilot study member suggested letting all non–Falun Gong individuals complete the HW2 without invitation from Falun Gong respondents. This would have distorted the research data and changed the focus of the research design, which was to compare two groups of respondents who are related or close to each other, and who share somewhat similar backgrounds, living or work environments, with the exception that one group practices Falun Gong and the other does not. Overall, the pilot study played an important role in the development phase and achieved its purpose in enabling useful feedback to refine the research tool. Pilot study members were sent an email thanking them for their involvement and contribution.

4.5 Instruments

There were two online surveys: HW1 for Falun Gong respondents; and HW2 for non–Falun Gong respondents. Both surveys comprised self-designed survey questions and the SF-36 Health Survey (McHorney et al., 1994; Ware Jr., 2008; Ware Jr. & Sherbourne, 1992). The online HW1 and HW2 surveys were in English language only. All responses were in English.

Chinese language versions (traditional and simplified form) were placed on the Falun Gong website only as a reference and guide for some Chinese-speaking respondents who might not be fluent in the English language. Accredited translators from the Australian National Accreditation Authority for Translators and Interpreters (NAATI) were used to translate the letter to respondents, the RIS, and the survey questions. Both Falun Gong and non–Falun Gong accredited NAATI translators were utilized in the translation process to ensure objectivity, accuracy, and to eliminate bias.

4.5.1 Self-designed survey questions

There were four sections in HW1 and three sections in HW2. The first two sections of both surveys consisted of self-designed questions. Section One collected the demographic details of respondents and Section Two their medical history and health status. In both surveys, the SF-36 Health Survey was the last section.

The difference between the two surveys was that HW1 had an extra section (Section Three) relating to Falun Gong practice. This extra section had 21 questions for Falun Gong respondents to self-report on their Falun Gong practice, which included changes in physical, emotional, and mental health, stress coping ability, relationship with significant others, and their attitude towards life since practicing Falun Gong. All questions asked for one answer except two, which requested Falun Gong respondents to select the three answers that best apply to their situation, from a range of eight options. The first of these questions was "What first attracted you to Falun Gong practice?" and the second was "How do you think Falun Gong practice has led to better health and wellness in your life?" Both questions had a sub-question with a text box for up to 2000 characters seeking a written qualitative response from respondents for 'other' explanations.

The rationale for collecting demographic data was to support the aim of Part A of this research, which was to obtain a demographic profile of Falun Gong practitioners from around the world. Besides the demographic data from surveys in mainland China (Author Unknown, 1998; Authors Unknown, 2002; Dan et al., 1998; Wang et al., 1998; Zhang & Xiao, 1996) and Taiwan (Lio et al., 2003), there were a few studies conducted in Canada and the United

States that presented a demographic profile of Falun Gong practitioners in certain regions of North America only (Authors Unknown, 2003a; Burgdoff, 2003; Lowe, 2003; Ownby, 2001, 2003b, 2008a; S. J. Palmer, 2003; Porter, 2003, 2005). To date, there has not been a demographic survey of Falun Gong practitioners in Australia and around the world.

Part A of this research aimed to address the following questions:
1. Who are the Falun Gong respondents, what are their ages, genders, and relationship statuses?
2. Where were they born and where are they residing?
3. What are their ethnicities, highest education level, occupations, and economic backgrounds?

Part B of this research investigated the health-wellness effects of Falun Gong as perceived by individuals who practice Falun Gong. It compared the medical history and general health-wellness statuses of Falun Gong respondents with non–Falun Gong respondents using a combination of self-designed survey questions and the Short Form (SF-36) Health Survey. Since this research investigated whether individuals who practice Falun Gong experience better health and wellness than those who do not, it was relevant to find out who these Falun Gong and non–Falun Gong individuals were, and the reasons for Falun Gong respondents to practice Falun Gong. This data could offer insight and understanding about Falun Gong and its practitioners.

4.5.2 Short Form (SF-36) Health Survey

The Short Form (SF-36) Health Survey was initially created to assess the general health status for the Medical Outcomes Study (Ware Jr., 2008; Ware Jr. & Sherbourne, 1992). (See Appendices 3 and 4 for Section 4 of HW1 and Section 3 of HW2 respectively.) It is a generic assessment suitable for measuring the health-wellness status of individuals in the general and diverse population (McHorney et al., 1994; Stanfeld et al., 1997; Ware Jr., 2008; Ware Jr. & Sherbourne, 1992).

This multi-purpose survey is simple to use and contains 36 items or questions. It is designed for self-administration for general, clinical, or non-clinical populations, and individuals from 14 years old to older adults (Author Unknown, 2008; Ware Jr. & Sherbourne, 1992). The SF-36 has been consistently tested and validated (Stanfeld et al., 1997; Ware Jr., 2000, 2008). There are approximately 4,000 publications on the use of the SF-36, making it one of the most widely used and documented general health assessment tools (Ware Jr., 2000, 2008). The SF-36 is suitable for online administration (Ware Jr., 2008), is versatile, and cost-free for research purposes.

The SF-36 was designed to assess eight health-wellness concepts (Author Unknown, 2008; Garratt et al., 1993; Jenkinson et al., 1993; Ware Jr., 2008; Ware Jr. & Sherbourne, 1992), which consisted of: 1) physical health (10 items); 2) social wellness (two items); 3) role limitations due to physical difficulty (four items); 4) role limitations due to emotional problems (three items); 5) mental health-wellness (five items); 6) vitality (four items); 7) physical pain (two items); and 8) perception of general health-wellness (six items) (Author Unknown, 2008; Garratt et al., 1993, p. 1441; Jenkinson et al., 1993, p. 1437; Stanfeld et al., 1997, p. 219; Ware Jr., 2008, p. 8; Ware Jr. & Sherbourne, 1992, p. 475). A scale of one indicated excellent health, or the best health outcome, not limited at all by any physical, mental, or emotional health concerns, while a higher scale indicated a poorer health outcome. Respondents were asked to choose what they thought was the best answer if they were unsure about how to answer any questions.

The eight health-wellness concepts included physical, mental, and emotional aspects, but not the spiritual dimension. This research was not designed to measure spiritual health-wellness or to investigate the role of spirituality in Falun Gong practice, making the SF-36 an appropriate choice of assessment instrument.

4.6 Respondents

There were two groups of respondents: Falun Gong and non–Falun Gong respondents. The non–Falun Gong respondents were invited by Falun Gong respondents to complete the HW2. They could be friends, colleagues, family members, relatives, or neighbors who had not practiced Falun Gong or any other similar meditative movement practices during the six months prior to completing the survey. The non–Falun Gong respondents were the comparison group.

There were two reasons for selecting the comparison group this way. The first was to maintain anonymity and avoid contact with the comparison respondents to eliminate or reduce researcher bias, response bias, and social desirability effects (Heerwegh, 2009; Tourangeau et al., 2003; VandenBos, 2007). The second reason was to make it more feasible to include non–Falun Gong respondents from multiple countries who might share similar characteristics with Falun Gong respondents, such as being in the same extended family (siblings, spouse, cousins, etc.), or friends from the same age group, or community, or work colleagues. These considerations, however, did not make the choice of an appropriate comparison group less problematic. Heppner et al. (1999) stated that there is no one "correct" (p. 387) way to structure a comparison group as long as the researcher understands the advantages and problems related to the choice of the comparison group. Their advice was for the researcher to bear in mind these limitations when analyzing, interpreting, and discussing the findings from the data (Heppner et al., 1999).

No maximum limit was placed on the number of respondents. However, there was a data collection cut-off date for completing the surveys. Participation was voluntary and respondents were not required to complete consent forms as the research was conducted using anonymous online surveys. This was in accordance with the HREC guidelines. No one was under any obligation to participate. Respondents were informed in the RIS that their responses would be kept confidential and unidentified in the data analysis and final research report. As requested by the HREC, a statement was included declaring that there was no absolute guarantee for the confidentiality or anonymity of information being transferred by email or Internet, and that every effort would be made to protect this.

The online surveys were open to all Falun Gong practitioners, their non–Falun Gong family members, and friends. Due to the severe persecution of Falun Gong practitioners in mainland China and various forms of intimidation in different countries by the CCP (H.R. Watch, 2002; Schechter, 2000; The Epoch Times, 2004; World Organization to Investigate the Persecution of Falun Gong, 2004), for security reasons and on recommendation from the HREC, a statement was added in the RIS and on the online surveys to caution potential respondents not to complete the survey if participating posed a security risk for them and their families.

4.6.1 Participation criteria

Participation and inclusion criteria for the Falun Gong and non–Falun Gong respondents were stated in the RIS. Failure to invite a non–Falun Gong respondent to complete HW2 or to choose one from the same age range would not disqualify Falun Gong respondents from participation. Many experienced practitioners, especially older Falun Gong practitioners, tend to have less social contact with non–Falun Gong individuals when all of their family members practice Falun Gong. This is comparable to ethnic, Christian, or other communities who tend to socialize within their own community groups (Court, 2007).

The rationale for the inclusion and exclusion criteria was to set limits to ensure collection of meaningful data and to minimize possible distortion and contamination of the data. Table 4.1 and Table 4.2 show the inclusion and exclusion criteria for Falun Gong and non–Falun Gong respondents respectively.

Table 4.1 Inclusion and exclusion criteria for Falun Gong respondents

Respondent	Inclusion Criteria	Exclusion Criteria
Falun Gong	Practice Falun Gong for at least 6 months; Engage in regular study of Falun Gong teachings; Engage in regular practice of Falun Gong exercises; Invite a non–Falun Gong family member, friend or colleague to do HW2.	Practice Falun Gong for less than 6 months; Not engaging in regular study of Falun Gong teachings; Not engaging in regular practice of Falun Gong exercises.

Table 4.2 Inclusion and exclusion criteria for non–Falun Gong respondents

Respondent	Inclusion Criteria	Exclusion Criteria
Non–Falun Gong	A friend or family member of a Falun Gong respondent; Not practicing Falun Gong in last 6 months; and Invited by a Falun Gong respondent to complete HW2.	Practicing Falun Gong in last 6 months; Practicing meditation, or other similar meditative movement practices, such as yoga, tai chi, and qigong in last 6 months.

4.7 Data collection phase

This phase involved transferring both HW1 and HW2 onto online format, liaising with pilot study members and the Falun Gong website postmaster, placing the surveys on the website, and disseminating the RIS to potential respondents to invite them to complete the surveys online. All items for HW1 and HW2 were manually transferred to the university's TellUS2 survey tool, checked, and then placed on the Australian Falun Dafa website, www.falunau.org. Once this process was successfully completed and the links for HW1 and HW2 were accessible, the URLs for the two online surveys were provided in the RIS.

Data collection commenced on Sunday, July 8, 2007 and ended on Monday, October 8, 2007. Respondents could click on the web links provided in the RIS to access and complete the surveys, or they could visit the Australian Falun Dafa website to complete the online surveys. Respondents were encouraged to complete the survey online, estimated to take about 20 minutes. Once data collection was completed, a thank you email was sent to the members of Falun Dafa associations, pilot study members, and respondents via group email lists.

4.7.1 Issues arising during data collection phase

There were several issues arising during the data collection period. The first was the adjustment of the time frame for data collection, which was originally set for five weeks. Later, it became apparent that the data collection period had to be extended to three months to provide more time for potential respondents from around the world to complete the online surveys. While most Falun Gong respondents were open to completing the online survey, finding a non–Falun Gong peer or family member was problematic for some Falun Gong respondents. Many experienced and also older practitioners had minimal social contact with non–Falun Gong individuals, especially when all of their family members practiced Falun Gong. Another query arose about whether the geographical location of the non–Falun Gong respondent had to be the same as the Falun Gong respondent. It was clarified that Falun Gong respondents could invite their relatives or friends from anywhere to complete HW2.

Although this research was an online survey, the researcher had indicated in the ethics protocol and the RIS that hard copy submissions would be possible. See Appendices 3 and 4 for the hard copy versions of the HW1 and HW2. There were 21 HW1 and 49 HW2 hard copy submissions received during the data collection period, although one of each of HW1 and HW2 were found to be incomplete and excluded. Additional hard copy submissions, received after the collection period, were also excluded.

4.8 Data processing and analysis phase

This is the third phase of the research process, which included reporting, analysis, interpretation, and presentation of the findings. After the cut-off date for data collection, a University of South Australia doctoral research assistant helped to manually enter the data from the hard copy submissions. The quantitative and qualitative data were automatically saved to Microsoft Excel documents, and then transferred manually, with each case identified via an anonymous identification number, to the Statistical Package for Social Sciences, Version 15 (SPSS) software program. There were 360 Falun Gong respondents and 230 non–Falun Gong respondents. The unequal sample size was not surprising given the difficulty some Falun Gong respondents had in finding a non–Falun Gong peer or family member to complete HW2.

Random audit checks were systematically conducted on the data entries for both groups during and on completion of the data transfer for quality control purposes and also to maintain data consistency and reliability. Horizontal column checks for every 30th and 20th respondent for HW1 and HW2 respectively were conducted. Vertical column scans were done for every 10th variable for both surveys as well as specifically checking the string variables. The data input for both groups were further scrutinized using SPSS descriptive frequency audit checks before data analysis commenced.

Missing data appeared to be randomly distributed. There were four noticeable cases of missing data in the Falun Gong group. Respondent 34 answered only the first three items and, for reasons unknown to the researcher, did not complete the rest of HW1. Respondent 250 completed Sections One and Two, and left Sections Three and Four blank, while the third one, Respondent 254, reported "Don't Know" for the first two questions and left the rest of Section Three (Meditation Practice) of HW1 blank. The fourth case, Respondent 166, left the entire HW1 blank. There were three missing cases with the non–Falun Gong group. Two non–Falun Gong respondents, Respondent 97 and 122, had missing data for the entire HW2, while the third one, Respondent 147, answered the first three questions for gender, age group, and relationship status, and for reasons unknown to the researcher, left the rest of the HW2 blank. The researcher treated all of these as missing data.

The quantitative and qualitative data have been reported and analyzed separately. The quantitative data was processed and analyzed using descriptive statistics. Items with single or short written responses were quantified, a process whereby qualitative data is converted into quantitative data (Sandelowski, 2000), and then transferred to SPSS database and analyzed using descriptive statistics. Written responses not quantified were analyzed and interpreted following a three-level categorizing or clustering procedure used in qualitative content analysis (Miles & Huberman, 1994), and adapted by other researchers (Graneheim & Lundman, 2004; Hanson et al., 2005; Sharif & Masoumi, 2005). Six items in Section One and five in Section Two of HW1 and HW2, as well as three items in Section Three of HW1 asked for written responses. All data from the HW1 and HW2 were reported according to the order of the items in the two surveys.

4.9 Summary

Chapter 4 provides an overview of the research design for this research. It has discussed the three main phases of the research and presented a flow chart to illustrate the entire process. The three phases comprised the development phase, data collection phase, and data processing and analysis phase. The research involved two parts: Part A to obtain a global demographic profile of Falun Gong practitioners; and Part B, the main component of the research, to investigate the health-wellness effects of Falun Gong as perceived by Falun Gong practitioners, and whether individuals who practice Falun Gong experience better health and wellness than those who do not practice Falun Gong. The study was designed as a descriptive cross-sectional online survey using a mixed methods approach that was mainly quantitative, with some qualitative content. The researcher was aware of the limitations of self-reporting in cross-sectional survey studies and issues around response bias when designing this survey, and undertook appropriate precautions. Further discussion of these issues is found in Chapter 9 of this book.

Chapter 5 now presents the findings of this research.

CHAPTER 5

Findings for
Falun Gong Respondents

5.1 Chapter overview

This chapter presents the findings for the first part of this research: Part A, the demographic profile of Falun Gong; and Part B, the investigation of the health-wellness effects of Falun Gong, as perceived by Falun Gong respondents. The findings are presented in four sections, based on HW1 survey for Falun Gong respondents. The first comprises the demographic profile of Falun Gong respondents, while the second pertains to the medical history, and health status of Falun Gong respondents. The third section focuses on the meditation practice, with 21 questions asking Falun Gong respondents about various aspects of their cultivation practice. The fourth section of the chapter presents the findings from the Short Form (SF-36) Health Survey. Findings from the two surveys revealed many similar demographic characteristics between Falun Gong and non–Falun Gong respondents. There were observed differences between the two groups in the self-reports of their medical history and general health-wellness status. Falun Gong respondents reported better health-wellness outcomes and were more likely to report excellent health and more positive self-perceptions of their health-wellness status than non–Falun Gong respondents.

5.2 Data reporting and analysis process

Data was individually transferred to the Statistical Package for Social Sciences (SPSS Version 15) software program. The quantitative and qualitative data were reported and analyzed using descriptive statistics and a three-level categorizing or clustering procedure (Miles & Huberman, 1994) as indicated in Chapter 3. All data are presented according to the order of the items in the two surveys. Tables, bar graphs, and pie charts were used to display the findings. The frequency and percentage calculations in tables and pie charts included missing data whereas bar charts produced by SPSS excluded missing data. Hence, overall total number of respondents in bar charts will not add up to 360 Falun Gong or 230 non–Falun Gong respondents respectively, unless the missing data is included, and this is reported either in the dissertation, or as a note below the bar charts (as in Chart 5.2) or the missing numbers are included in the pie chart (as in Chart 5.1). All tables and charts were checked for their frequency and percentage totals.

The larger number of respondents in this research compared to previous Falun Gong studies in Canada and the United States (Burgdoff, 2003; Lau, 2001; Q. Li et al., 2005; Lowe, 2003; Ownby, 2003b, 2008a; S. J. Palmer, 2003; Porter, 2003) and their international variance posed challenges for what was intended to be a simple global demographic data report and analysis. For example, conversion of diverse local currencies to the Australian dollar created difficulties in interpreting respondents' health costs and living standards, and therefore it was unrealistic to display the data of some items in any visual form.

5.3 Findings for the Falun Gong respondents

5.3.1 Section 1: Demographic profile

The demographic profile of Falun Gong respondents is presented across their gender, age range, relationship status, ethnicity, country of birth and residence, first language, highest education level, occupation, and gross annual household income. There were a total of 360 Falun Gong respondents. Overall, the sample size largely comprised young married females, who were tertiary educated with professional occupations, and whose first language was not English.

5.3.1.1 Gender distribution

There were more female than male Falun Gong respondents as illustrated in Chart 5.1.

Chart 5.1 Gender distribution of Falun Gong respondents

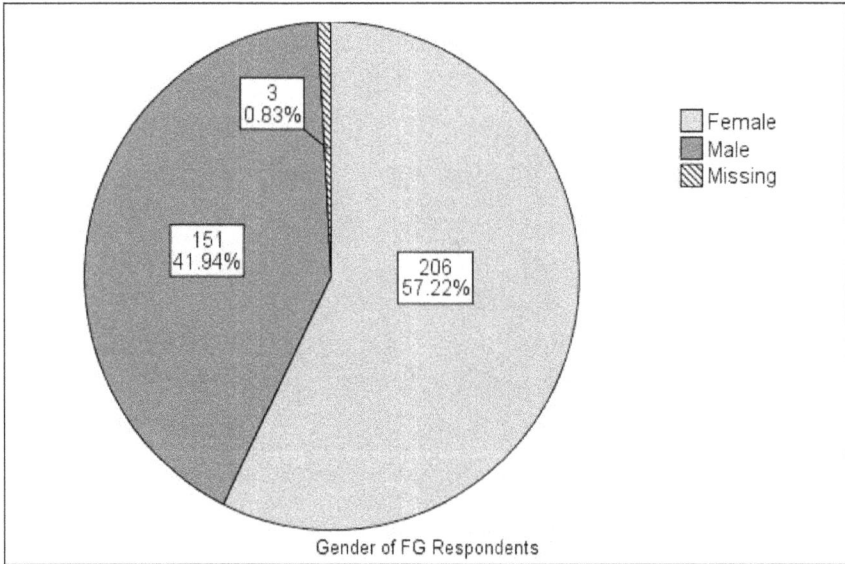

Gender of FG Respondents

5.3.1.2 Age range

The Falun Gong respondents were asked to identify their age within seven ranges as shown in Chart 5.2. Falun Gong respondents aged 30 to 39 years comprised the largest age range group with the youngest age range of less than 20 years containing the smallest number of respondents. The average age of Falun Gong respondents was located between the 30 to 39 years of age range and 40 to 49 years of age range.

Chart 5.2 Age range of Falun Gong respondents

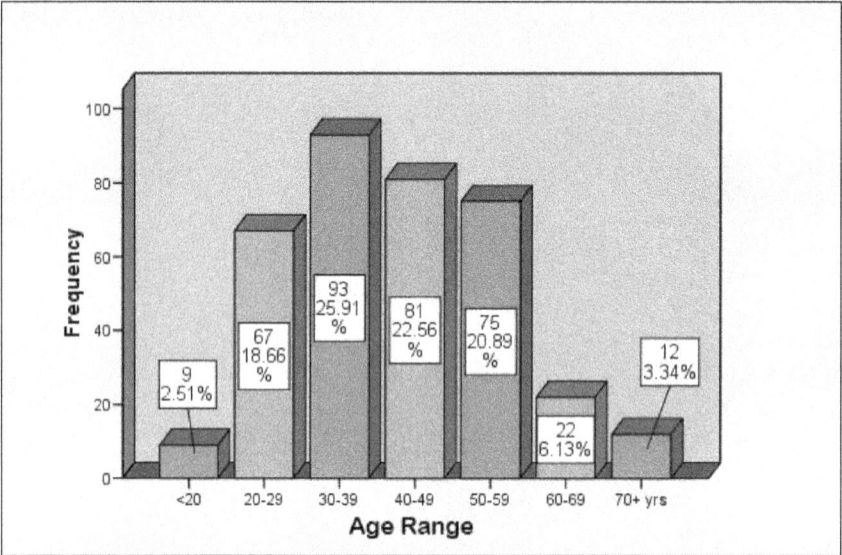

Note: Missing=1

5.3.1.3 Relationship status

The Falun Gong respondents were asked to indicate their relationship status according to a range of five options. As shown in Chart 5.3, nearly two-thirds of Falun Gong respondents (61%, n=218, missing=2) were married, with only five respondents in a de facto relationship.

Chart 5.3 Relationship status of Falun Gong respondents

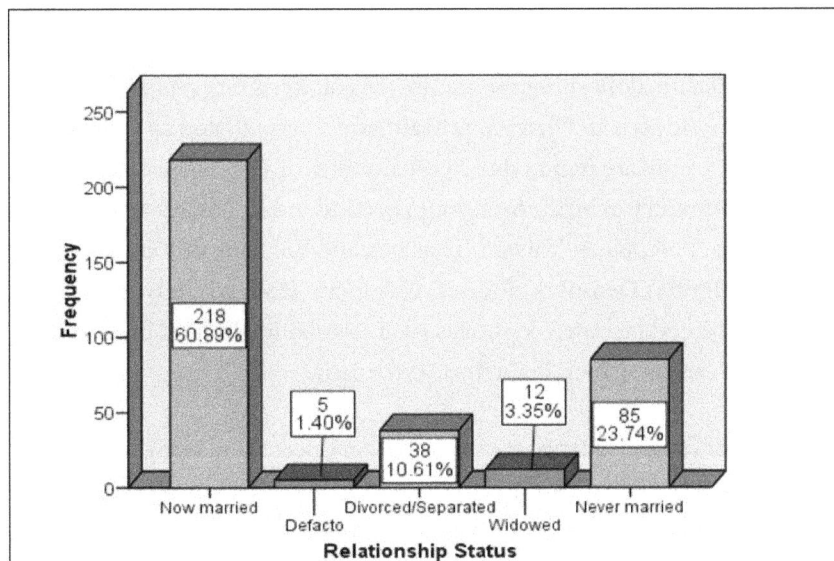

5.3.1.4 Ethnicity

The Falun Gong respondents were able to identify their ethnicity. Their ethnicities were diverse and wide-ranging, with 37 identified in total. These included one each from Africa, Albania, an Australian Aborigine, two Maori, three Native North American Indians, two Turks, three Filipinos, four Jews, as well as Russian, Polish, and Spanish respondents. Others identified themselves from the Mediterranean and Scandinavian regions, India, and different parts of Asia, such as Japan, Korea, Malaysia, Indonesia, Singapore, and Thailand. Some respondents identified themselves as Anglo-Celtic, Chinese-Vietnamese, Chinese-Korean, Eurasian, Hispanic, Papuan New Guinea/Australian, and Russian Slav. Chinese formed the largest group (47.3%, n=170). Approximately a quarter of Falun Gong respondents (24%, n=86) identified themselves as Caucasians, with others as Anglo-Celtic (n=1), Scandinavian (n=1), American (n=4), Australian (n=26), Canadian (n=1), or New Zealander (n=1). Because of the ethnic diversity, it was unrealistic to display this data in any visual form.

5.3.1.5 Country of birth

As identification of country of birth was not prescribed in the survey, the researcher classified the different nominated countries into regions for easier reporting, as shown in Chart 5.4. Mainland China (listed as China) was classified as a separate region due to the number of respondents identifying this as their country of birth. Asia comprised Indonesia, Malaysia, Singapore, Japan, Korea, Philippines, Taiwan, Thailand, and Vietnam. Europe comprised Austria, Belgium, Denmark, France, Germany, Holland, Italy, Spain, and Sweden. "Others" included countries such as Albania, India, Libya, Poland, the Mediterranean, Israel, Mauritius, and Russia.

Overall, 45 different countries of birth were identified. Falun Gong respondents born in mainland China comprised the largest number (28%, n=97, missing=8), with the second highest number born in Asia (24%, n=86) and the third highest, those born in Australia and New Zealand (19%, n=68), as shown in Chart 5.4.

Chart 5.4 Country of birth of Falun Gong respondents

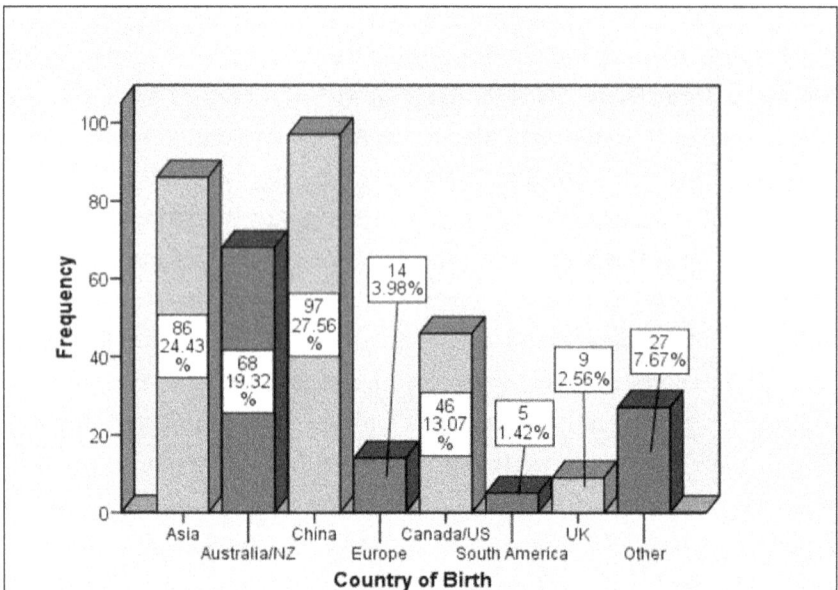

5.3.1.5 Country of residence

As with ethnicity and country of origin, country of residence was not prescribed for respondents. The countries identified were classified as for country of birth, indicated in Chart 5.5. Falun Gong respondents live in diverse countries and regions around the world with 29 different countries and regions identified. Despite this diversity, 75% of Falun Gong respondents (n=268, missing=4) resided in two main regions, Australia and New Zealand, and Canada and the U.S.

Chart 5.5 Country of residence of Falun Gong respondents

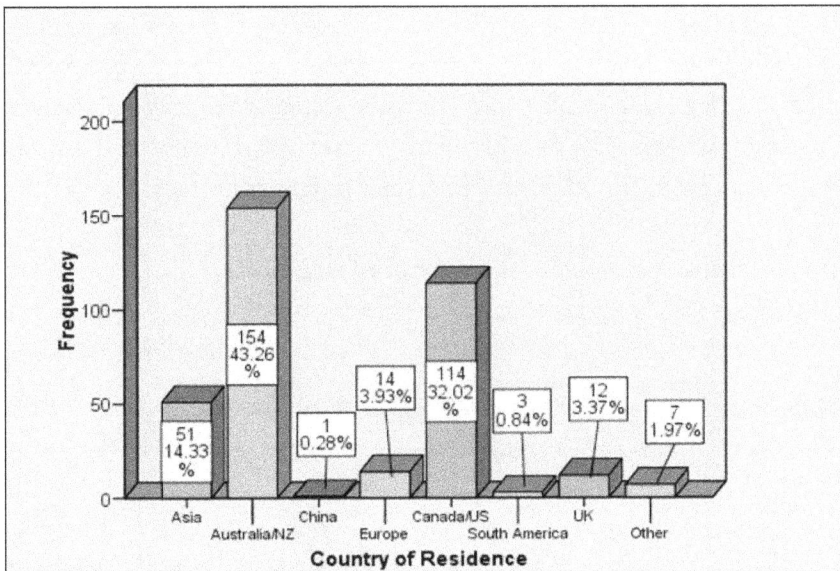

5.3.1.7 First language

The Falun Gong respondents were asked to indicate if English was their first language. The term first language was defined as "the language you grew up with as a child." English was the first language for 35% of Falun Gong respondents (n=128), while 63% (n=226) indicated it was not. Almost half of the Falun Gong respondents (44%, n=164) reported either Mandarin or Chinese dialects, such as Cantonese, Hakka, and Shanghainese, as their first language.

The diversity of Falun Gong respondents' country of origin was reflected in the variety of languages they spoke. These included an Australian Aboriginal language, North American Native Navajo language, African Igbo language, Marathi language, as well as a variety of Asian, European and Eastern European languages. These included Bahasa Indonesia, Bahasa Malaysia, Japanese, Korean, Tagalog, Thai, Vietnamese, Albanian, Creole, Croatian, Dutch, French, German, Greek, Hebrew, Hungarian, Italian, Lebanese, Norwegian, Polish, Portuguese Spanish, and Turkish.

5.3.1.8 Highest education level of Falun Gong respondents

The Falun Gong respondents were asked to identify their highest level of education based on five provided options as shown in Chart 5.6. Over 63% of Falun Gong respondents (n=224, missing=5) indicated they had tertiary qualifications, with 30% (n=107) having a master's, PhD or doctoral degree. Respondents were not asked to specify their programs of study.

Chart 5.6 Highest education level of Falun Gong respondents

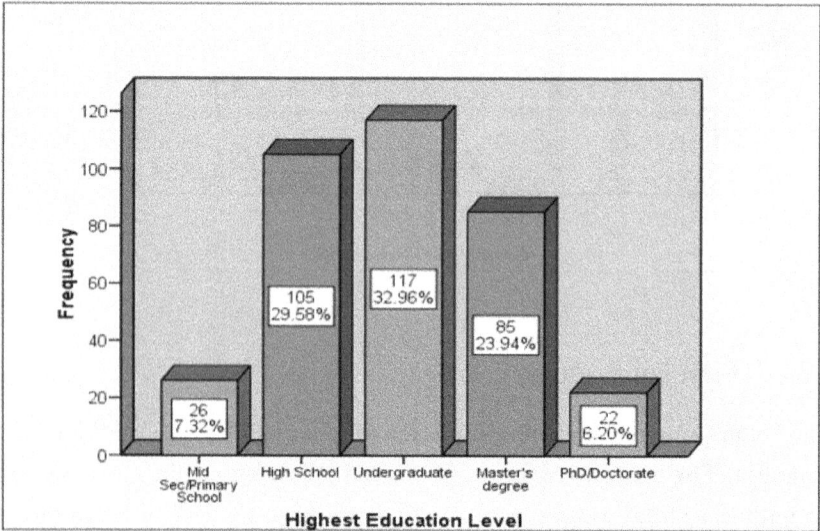

5.3.1.9 Occupations

The Falun Gong respondents were able to indicate their occupation. The Australian and New Zealand Standard Classification of Occupations (ANZSCO), as provided by the Australian Bureau of Statistics (ABS) and Statistics New Zealand (SNZ) (Australian Bureau of Statistics & Statistics New Zealand, 2006) was used to categorize the responses. Appendix 5 details the major categories and subcategories of occupations as derived from the ABS (2006) and SNZ (2006).

Falun Gong respondents reported a wide range of occupations, ranging from unemployment, being a student, skilled and unskilled labor work to professional, executive and senior administrative positions. Arts, media, social sciences, miscellaneous professionals, and business/computer information technology professionals comprised the largest number of respondents (15.25%, n=54). Clerical, sales, administrative and service workers, and retired/home duties had the second largest number of Falun Gong respondents, with equal numbers of respondents respectively (12.15%, n=43). Skilled and unskilled laborers, and the unemployed comprised the smallest categories, with less than five percent of Falun Gong respondents (n=17).

Chart 5.7 indicates the frequency and percentage distribution across the major categories of occupations of Falun Gong respondents.

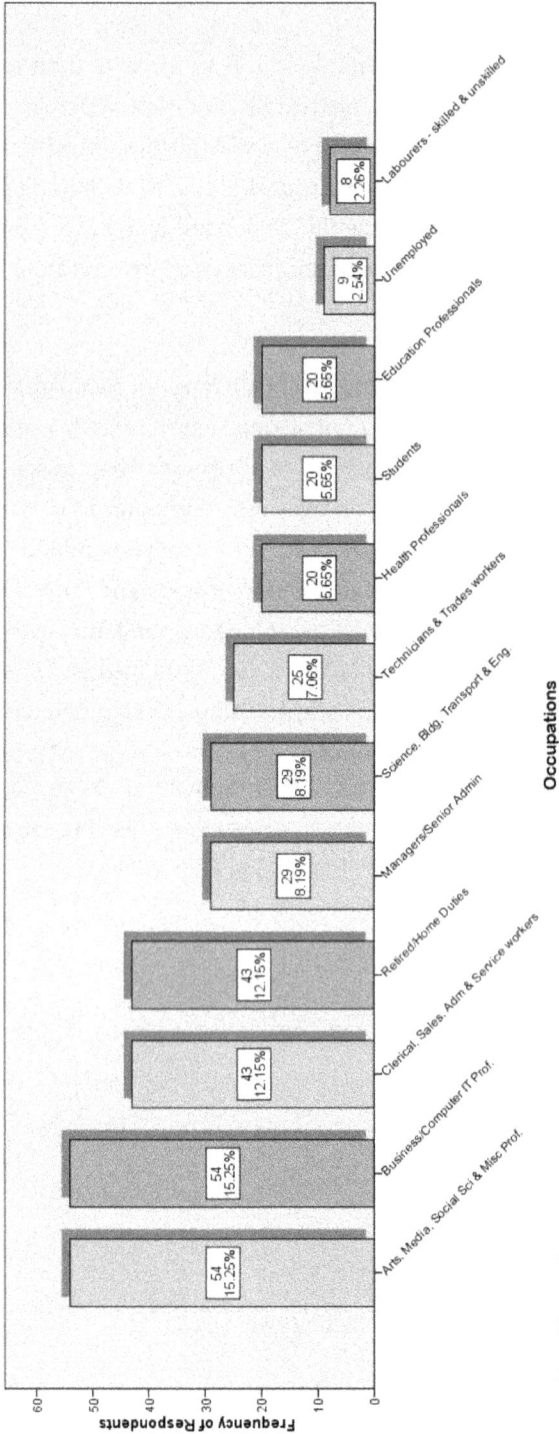

Chart 5.7 Occupations of Falun Gong respondents

Note: Missing=6

5.3.1.10 Gross annual income

The Falun Gong respondents were lastly asked to indicate their gross annual household income in their local currency. It was intended to convert the reported incomes to Australian dollars. However, currency conversion to Australian dollars rendered it impossible to make any interpretation or comparison because of the huge gaps and extreme differences in the standards and costs of living in different countries. It was therefore decided to not report on this item for both Falun Gong and non–Falun Gong respondents.

5.3.2 Section 2: Medical history and health status

Section 2 of the survey comprised 13 items asking Falun Gong respondents about their medical history, number of medical consultations, reasons for medical consultations, medication intake history, medical and health expenses, cigarette smoking, alcohol consumption, and recreational drug use habits. Overall, Falun Gong respondents indicated they were healthy individuals with very healthy lifestyle habits. Most of them did not visit medical practitioners, took no medications and spent very little money on medical and health expenses. They were typically non-smokers and did not drink alcohol or use recreational drugs.

5.3.2.1 Visits to medical practitioners

The Falun Gong respondents were asked to report the number of visits they had made to a physician during the previous six months. The majority had not consulted a medical practitioner with few respondents seeking medical help more than seven to nine times, as shown in Table 5.1.

Table 5.1 Number of visits to a medical doctor by Falun Gong respondents

Number of Medical Visits	Frequency	Percent
None	316	87.8
1-3 times	30	8.3
4-6 times	5	1.4
7-9 times	3	0.8
> 10 times	0	0
Missing	6	1.7
Total	360	100.0

5.3.2.2 Reason for medical visits

The qualitative data for this item is reported in Chapter 7.

5.3.2.3 Use of medication and health supplements

The Falun Gong respondents were provided with a range of medication and health supplement options and asked to identify all that applied to their situation. The majority (95%, n=341) reported not using any form of medication or health supplements, as shown in Table 5.2.

Table 5.2 Use of medication and health supplements by Falun Gong respondents

Options	Description of Items	Frequency	Percent
1	None	341	94.7
2	Prescription drugs (medical)	7	1.9
3	Over the counter drugs, e.g. Panadol, Aspirin	1	0.3
4	Chinese herbal remedies	0	0
5	Western herbal remedies	1	0.3
6	Homeopathic remedies	1	0.3
7	Vitamins and health supplements	5	1.4
Missing		4	1.1
Total		360	100.0

5.3.2.4 Medical and health expenses

The Falun Gong respondents were invited to report all their medical and health expenses, including prescriptions, herbal remedies, supplements, naturopathic, vitamins and health supplements, and so on during the past six months prior to the survey. Total costs were requested in local currency with the intention of converting all reported expenses to Australian dollars. Currency conversion to the Australian dollar, however, made it impossible to interpret or compare findings because of the differences in the standards and costs of living in different countries. The majority of Falun Gong respondents (92%, n=330) stated that they did not spend any money on medical and health expenses. Only eight percent of Falun Gong respondents (n=30) reported spending money on health and medical expenses, with some reporting health insurance premiums as their only health expense.

5.3.2.5 Cigarette smoking, alcohol intake, and recreational drug use

The Falun Gong respondents were requested to report whether they were involved in substance use, such as cigarette smoking, alcohol consumption, and recreational drug use. They were asked to state the amount of substance use and if they had plans to stop using it. Falun Gong respondents were typically non-smokers who did not drink alcohol or use recreational drugs.

5.3.2.5.1 Cigarette smoking by Falun Gong respondents

Nearly all Falun Gong respondents (98%, n=352) reported not smoking any tobacco cigarettes as illustrated in Chart 5.8. Only five Falun Gong respondents reported smoking cigarettes and two of them planned to stop.

Chart 5.8 Cigarette smoking by Falun Gong respondents

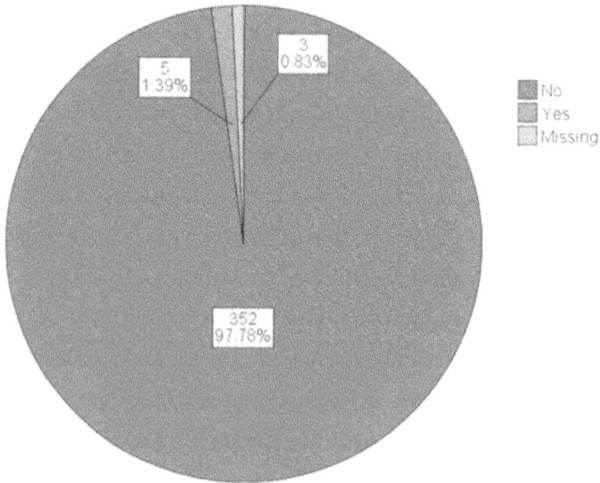

5.3.2.5.2 Alcohol consumption by Falun Gong respondents

Similarly, almost all Falun Gong respondents (97%, n=349) reported not consuming any form of alcohol. Only eight Falun Gong respondents did report consuming alcohol across a range of amounts. Chart 5.9 shows the frequency and percentage distribution of alcohol consumption by Falun Gong respondents.

Chart 5.9 Alcohol consumption by Falun Gong respondents

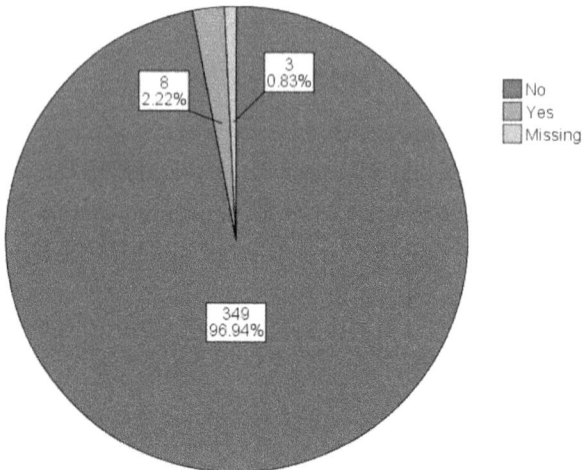

5.3.2.5.3 Recreational drug use

Almost all Falun Gong respondents (98.6%, n=355) reported not taking any recreational drugs. Only one Falun Gong respondent reported drug use, but this was not a recreational drug.

Chart 5.10 Recreational drug use by Falun Gong respondents

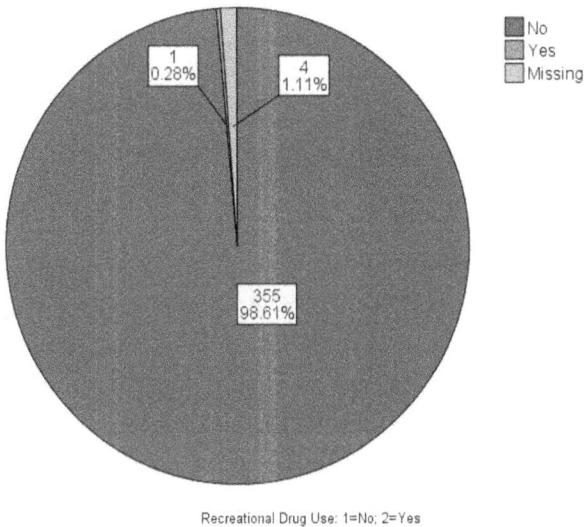

Recreational Drug Use: 1=No; 2=Yes

5.3.3 Section 3: Meditation practice

Section Three of HW1 comprised 21 questions asking Falun Gong respondents to: define Falun Gong; identify characteristics of their practice; and changes, if any, in physical, mental and emotional health, stress coping ability, relationship with others, and their attitude towards life since practicing Falun Gong. These questions were only for Falun Gong respondents pertaining to their practice. See Appendix 3 for Section 3 of the HW1. Falun Gong respondents were asked to report any pre-existing medical condition(s) and to compare this with after commencing Falun Gong. They were also asked to indicate what first attracted them to Falun Gong and what they thought had led to better health and wellness in their life.

Overall, the respondents were veteran Falun Gong practitioners. Mr. Li Hongzhi (2001b) used the term "veteran" (p. 41) to refer to more experienced Falun Gong practitioners who have been practicing for a number of years and have a sound understanding of Falun Gong teachings. Most Falun Gong respondents reported engaging in regular 'Fa study' and practice of the exercises. Fa study refers to the study of Falun Gong teachings by oneself or in groups (H. Li, 1996, 1999, 2007a, 2007b, 2008). Falun Gong respondents reported perceived significant improvements in various aspects of their life and being initially attracted to Falun Gong for different reasons besides the teachings of Falun Gong, their belief in predestined relationships or *yuanfen,* and the search for meaning in life. These are presented in Chapter 7 on written comments from the qualitative data reporting.

5.3.3.1 Description of Falun Gong

The Falun Gong respondents were asked to choose the most appropriate option to describe Falun Gong. Almost all Falun Gong respondents (98%, n=351) selected "Also known as Falun Dafa, it is an advanced cultivation practice based on Truthfulness, Compassion and Forbearance." Two respondents (0.6%) described Falun Gong as "a type of qigong," while another two indicated "Don't know." No respondent identified Falun Gong as a form of religion, a Taoist or Buddhist sect.

5.3.3.2 Most important aspect of Falun Gong practice

The majority of Falun Gong respondents identified "Study Falun Gong teachings" as the most important aspect of Falun Gong practice. Maintaining a positive attitude or having a righteous state of mind was rated second most important as indicated in Table 5.3.

Table 5.3 Most important aspect of Falun Gong practice

Description of Options	Frequency	Percent
Practice exercises	10	2.8
Study Falun Gong teachings	329	91.4
Maintain positive attitude	15	4.2
Experience sharing conference	0	0
Don't know	3	0.8
Missing	3	0.8
Total	360	100.0

5.3.3.3 Number of years of Falun Gong practice

The Falun Gong respondents were asked to indicate the number of years they had been practicing Falun Gong. Over half of the respondents (54%, n=194, missing=6) were veteran practitioners who reported practicing Falun Gong from six to more than ten years, as shown in Chart 5.11.

Chart 5.11 Number of years of Falun Gong practice

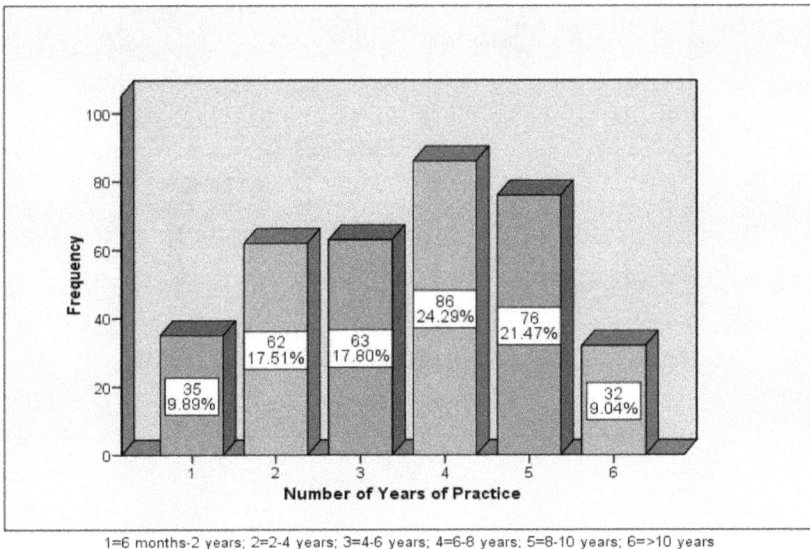

1=6 months-2 years; 2=2-4 years; 3=4-6 years; 4=6-8 years; 5=8-10 years; 6=>10 years

5.3.3.4 Frequency of Falun Gong practice

The Falun Gong respondents were asked to indicate the frequency of their exercise practice each week according to four options: once a week; two to three times a week; four to five times a week; or daily practice. Respondents reported practicing the exercises on a regular basis, with more than half of respondents (58%, n=203) engaging in daily exercise practice or at least four to five times a week.

5.3.3.5 Time spent on Falun Gong practice

The Falun Gong respondents were asked to report the time spent on Falun Gong practice. Forty-one percent of Falun Gong respondents (n=144, missing=7) indicated an hour of practice for each session. Over two-thirds (68%, n=239) spent one hour to one-and-a-half hours practicing Falun Gong exercises during each session, as indicated in Chart 5.12

Chart 5.12 Time spent on Falun Gong practice

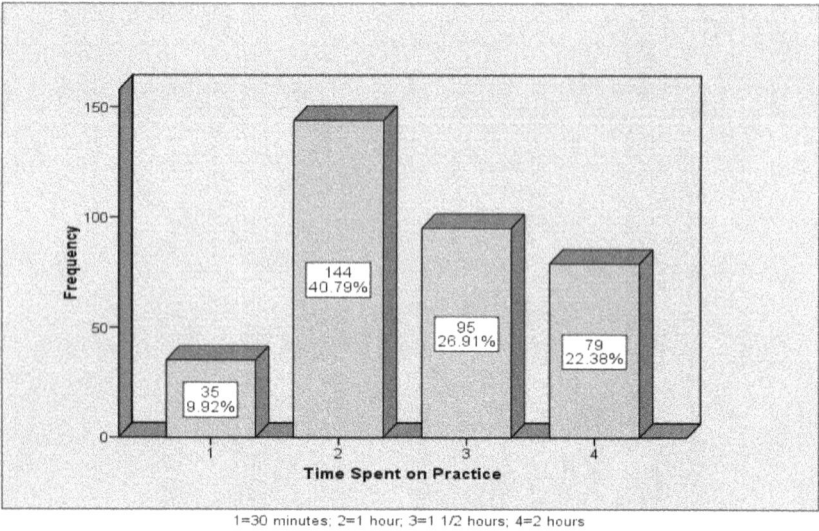

1=30 minutes; 2=1 hour; 3=1 1/2 hours; 4=2 hours

5.3.3.6 Frequency of Fa study

The Falun Gong respondents were provided with four options to report the frequency of Fa study they engaged in each week. Nearly three-quarters of Falun Gong respondents (72%, n=253, missing=7) engaged in daily Fa study as shown in Chart 5.13.

Chart 5.13 Frequency of Fa study

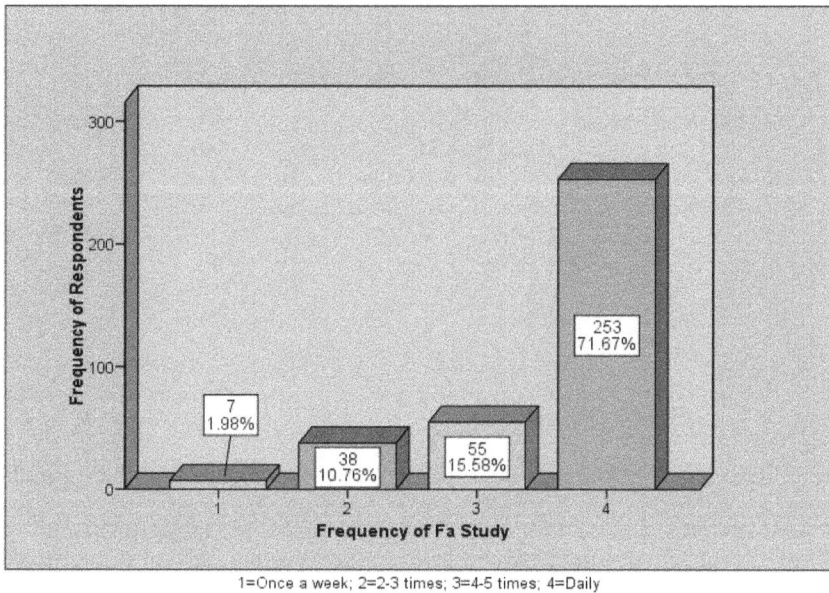

1=Once a week; 2=2-3 times; 3=4-5 times; 4=Daily

5.3.3.7 Total time spent on Fa study

The Falun Gong respondents were asked to nominate the total amount of time spent on Fa study each week according to a range of six options, as shown in Chart 5.14. Nearly all Falun Gong respondents (99%, n=349, missing=11) reported spending time each week on Fa study. Almost two-thirds of Falun Gong respondents (62%, n=224) reported spending six to fifteen hours each week on Fa study.

Chart 5.14 Total time spent on Fa study

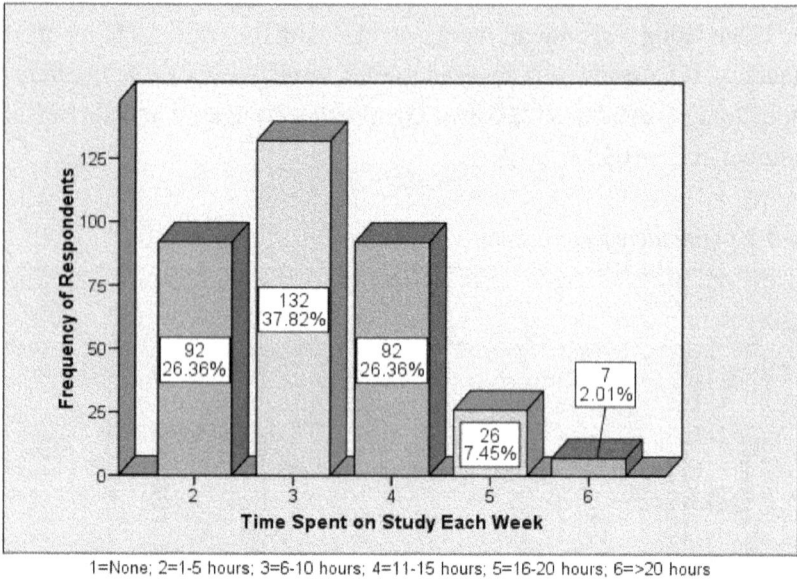

1=None; 2=1-5 hours; 3=6-10 hours; 4=11-15 hours; 5=16-20 hours; 6=>20 hours

5.3.3.8 Change in physical health

The Falun Gong respondents were asked to rate any change in physical health across five options (see Appendix 3 for the HW1), ranging from significantly worse, slightly worse, no difference, slightly improved, to significantly improved. The majority of respondents (98%, n=346) reported perceived improvement in their physical health since starting Falun Gong practice. Two Falun Gong respondents (0.6%) indicated a worsening of their physical health.

5.3.3.9 Change in mental and emotional health

The Falun Gong respondents were provided with five options to rate any change in mental and emotional health since commencing Falun Gong practice, as shown in Chart 5.15. The majority of Falun Gong respondents (93%, n=325, missing=10) reported a perceived significant improvement in their mental and emotional health. Two respondents (0.6%) indicated a worsening of their mental and emotional health.

Chart 5.15 Change in mental and emotional health

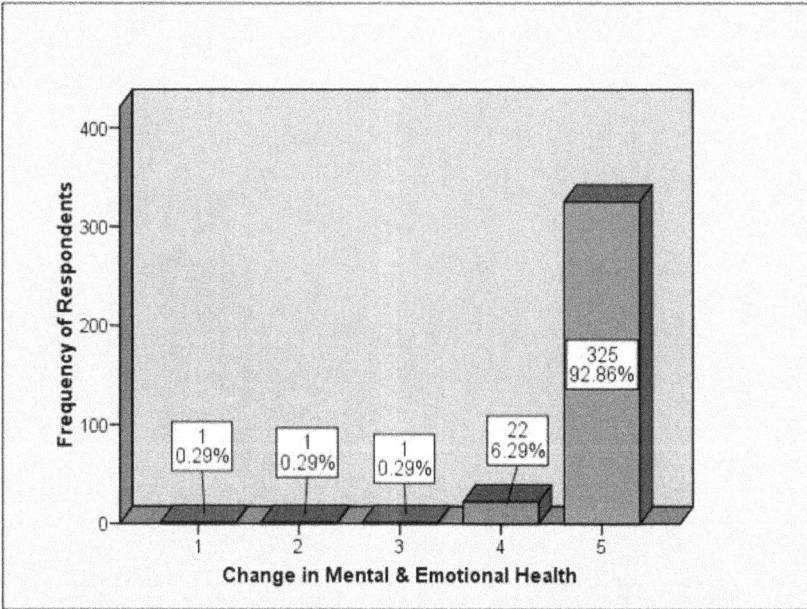

1=Significantly worse; 2=Slightly worse; 3=No difference; 4=Slightly improved; 5=Significantly improved

5.3.3.10 Change in stress coping ability

The Falun Gong respondents were given five options to rate any change in their stress coping ability since starting Falun Gong as shown in Chart 5.16. The majority of Falun Gong respondents reported perceived significant improvement in their stress coping ability. Two respondents (0.6%, missing=8) indicated a worsening of their stress coping ability.

Chart 5.16 Change in stress coping ability

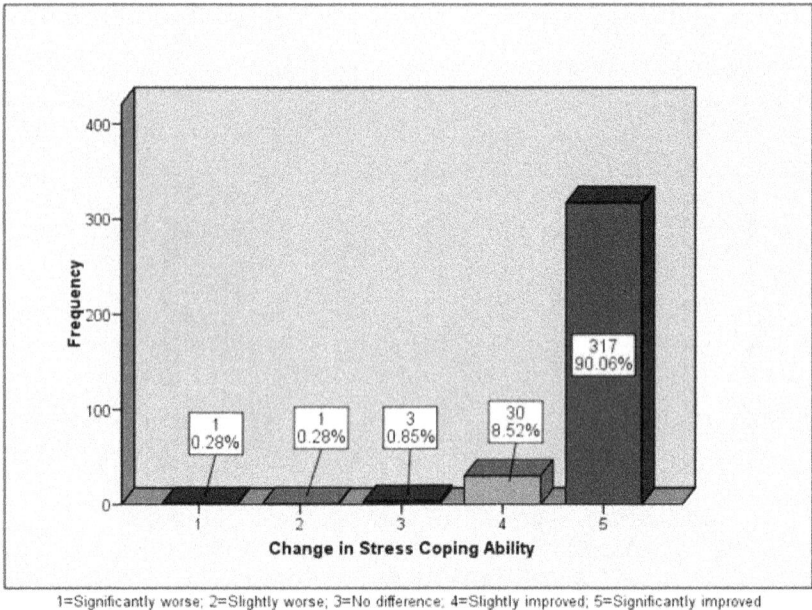

1=Significantly worse; 2=Slightly worse; 3=No difference; 4=Slightly improved; 5=Significantly improved

5.3.3.11 Change in relationship with significant others

The Falun Gong respondents were asked to rate any change in relationship with significant others across five options. Findings indicated that 91% of Falun Gong respondents (n=325) reported a perceived improvement in their relationship with significant others since practicing Falun Gong. Eight respondents (2.2%) did indicate a deterioration of their relationship with significant people in their life since practicing Falun Gong.

5.3.3.12 Change in attitude towards life

The Falun Gong respondents were provided with five options, as illustrated in Chart 5.17, to rate any change in their attitude towards life since practicing Falun Gong. Nearly all Falun Gong respondents (99%, n=351, missing=6) reported a perceived improvement in their attitude towards life. One respondent indicated "no difference" in their attitude towards life, while another two (0.6%) reported deterioration in their attitude towards life.

Chart 5.17 Change in attitude towards life

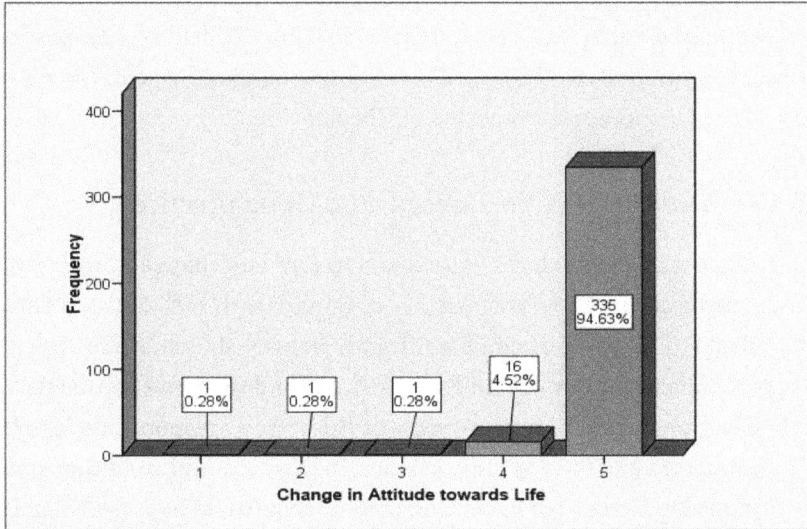

1=Significantly worse; 2=Slightly worse; 3=No difference; 4=Slightly improved; 5=Significantly improved

5.3.3.13 Quit tobacco smoking after Falun Gong practice

The Falun Gong respondents who smoked tobacco cigarettes prior to practicing Falun Gong were asked if they stopped smoking after starting Falun Gong practice. Seventy-seven percent of Falun Gong respondents (n=276) indicated this was "Not Applicable" to them. Of those (19%, n=68) who smoked tobacco cigarettes before starting Falun Gong practice, 82.3% (n=56) of them reported that they quit their smoking habit after they began Falun Gong.

5.3.3.14 Stop alcohol consumption after Falun Gong practice

The Falun Gong respondents who consumed alcohol prior to practicing Falun Gong were asked if they stopped drinking alcohol after starting Falun Gong practice. Nearly half of respondents (47%, n=169) indicated this was "Not Applicable" to them. Of those (48%, n=174) who reported consuming alcohol prior to Falun Gong practice, 97% (n=168) of them indicated that they stopped alcohol consumption after starting Falun Gong practice. Only six reported not giving up alcohol consumption.

5.3.3.15 Medical condition before Falun Gong practice

Just over half of Falun Gong respondents (53%, n=189) had no pre-existing medical condition(s), while 46% (n=164) indicated that they did. Details of their written responses are reported in Chapter 7.

5.3.3.16 Medical condition since Falun Gong practice

The Falun Gong respondents were asked to rate any change in their pre-existing medical condition(s) across five options. Nearly 60% of Falun Gong respondents (n=211) reported, "Significantly improved," while 5.3% (n=19) indicated, "Slightly improved" in their medical condition after commencing Falun Gong practice. About two-thirds of Falun Gong respondents (64.3%, n=230) reported a perceived improvement in their medical condition since practicing Falun Gong. One Falun Gong respondent (0.3%) indicated "Slightly worse," while another reported "Significantly worse" since commencing Falun Gong practice. Analysis of the data (to be discussed in Chapter 9) revealed that the same Falun Gong respondent (R27), a veteran practitioner, reported a significant worsening of their medical condition across all the five health-wellness dimensions.

This completes the quantitative content reporting for Section 3 of HW1 for Falun Gong respondents. The qualitative data for Items 38 and 42 to 45 will be reported in Chapter 7.

5.3.4 Section 4: Short Form (SF-36) Health Survey

This section presents findings from the Short Form (SF-36) Health Survey, comprising 36 items seeking self-reports from Falun Gong respondents about their general, physical, mental, and emotional health status, how they felt and how well they were able to perform their normal daily activities. The 36 items are reported individually or in clusters, where appropriate, to reflect the eight health-wellness concepts, summarized in Chapter 4 (Research Design). Overall, Falun Gong respondents reported not being limited by ill health to perform most of their normal daily and social activities, with more than half (53%, n=192) reporting excellent general health status. Most Falun Gong respondents perceived themselves as physically, mentally and emotionally very healthy, with a positive and optimistic outlook of their health-wellness status.

5.3.4.1 General health status

The Falun Gong respondents were asked to indicate their general health status according to five options, as shown in Chart 5.18. Most Falun Gong respondents (88%, n=317, missing=4) reported either excellent or very good general health status. One respondent rated poor general health status.

Chart 5.18 General health status of Falun Gong respondents

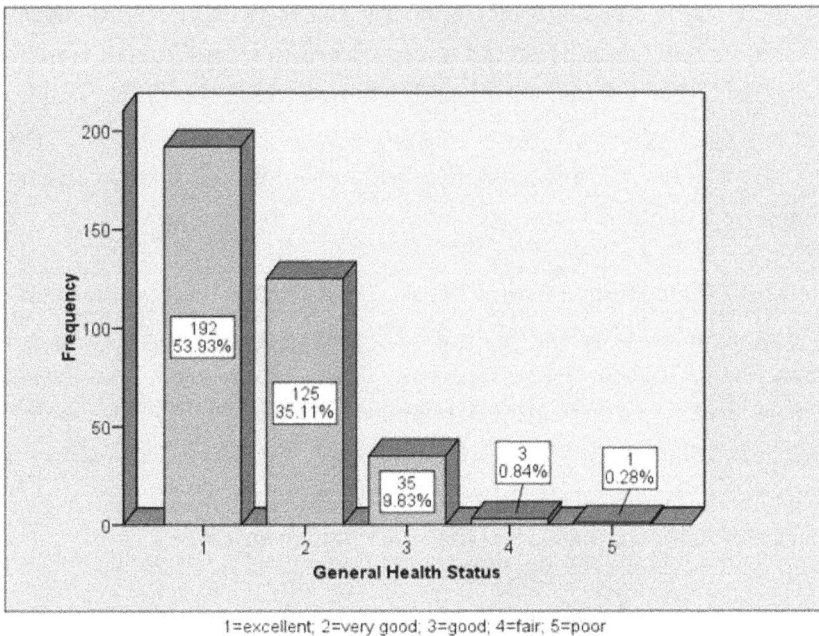

1=excellent; 2=very good; 3=good; 4=fair; 5=poor

5.3.4.2 General health one year ago

The Falun Gong respondents were provided with five options to indicate their general health compared to one year ago. Twenty-eight percent of Falun Gong respondents (n=101) were "much better" than a year ago while 29% (n=105) reported being "somewhat better." One respondent (0.3%) reported being "much worse" in terms of general health than a year ago.

5.3.4.3 How health limits daily activities

This subsection reports 10 items from the SF-36 Survey that assess physical health relating to daily activities and normal physical functioning for a typical day. Respondents were given three options to indicate whether their health had limited them from a range of activities that they might do during a typical day.

Seventy-three percent of Falun Gong respondents (n=261) reported that their health was not limited at all in terms of vigorous activities, such as running or lifting heavy objects. The majority (93%, n=333) reported not being limited by their health in performing moderate activities like moving a small table or using a domestic vacuum cleaner. Similarly, 93% of Falun Gong respondents (n=333) reported their health did not restrict them from lifting or carrying groceries. When asked if their health had restricted them from climbing several flights of stairs, 87% of Falun Gong respondents (n=314) reported "no" and 93% (n=335) reported their health did not limit them at all from climbing one flight of stairs.

Most Falun Gong respondents (91%, n=328) stated that their health had not limited them at all from bending, kneeling or stooping. Likewise, 91% of Falun Gong respondents (n=326) reported their health did not limit them at all from walking more than a mile. Ninety-three percent (n=333) reported their health did not limit them from walking several blocks. The majority of Falun Gong respondents (95%, n=342) stated they were not limited at all in terms of walking one block, bathing or dressing themselves.

Chart 5.4 displays the frequency and percentage distribution of Falun Gong respondents for each of these 10 items.

Table 5.4 How health limits daily activities of Falun Gong respondents

	Vigorous Activities		Moderate Activities		Lift or Carry Groceries		Climb Several Stairs		Climb One Flight of Stairs		Bend, Kneel or Stoop		Walk More than a Mile		Walk Several Blocks		Walk One Block		Bathe or Dress yourself	
	F	%	F	%	F	%	F	%	F	%	F	%	F	%	F	%	F	%	F	%
1	261	72.5	333	92.5	333	92.5	314	87.2	335	93.1	328	91.1	326	90.6	333	92.5	342	95.0	343	95.3
2	78	21.7	16	4.4	15	4.2	38	10.6	11	3.1	20	5.6	21	5.8	17	4.7	7	1.9	8	2.2
3	16	4.4	8	2.2	7	1.9	3	0.8	5	1.4	6	1.7	6	1.7	4	1.1	5	1.4	4	1.1
Sub-Total	355	98.6	357	99.2	355	98.6	355	98.6	351	97.5	354	98.3	353	98.1	354	98.3	354	98.3	355	98.6
(M)	5	1.4	3	0.8	5	1.4	5	1.4	9	2.5	6	1.7	7	1.9	6	1.7	6	1.7	5	1.4
Total	360	100	360	100	360	100	360	100	360	100	360	100	360	100	360	100	360	100	360	100

1=Not Limited at all; 2=Yes, Limited a Little; 3=Yes, Limited a Lot; F=Frequency; M=Missing; %=Percentage of Falun Gong Respondents
For visual clarity, gridlines are added.

5.3.4.4 Problems due to physical health

This subsection reports four items from the SF-36 that measure the physical aspect of the eight health-wellness concepts. Falun Gong respondents were asked to report whether they had any problems with their work or other regular daily activities due to their physical health. Table 5.5 shows the frequency and percentage distribution of Falun Gong respondents for the four items.

Table 5.5 Problems with work due to physical health (Falun Gong respondents)

	Reduce Work Time		Do Less than You Like		Limited in Work or Activities		Difficulty Doing Work	
	F	%	F	%	F	%	F	%
No	342	95.0	331	91.9	337	93.6	40	94.4
Yes	14	3.9	23	6.4	15	4.2	15	4.2
Missing	4	1.1	6	1.7	8	2.2	5	1.4
Total	360	100	360	100	360	100	360	100

F=Frequency

The majority of Falun Gong respondents reported having no problems with their work or daily activities due to their physical health. Overall, Falun Gong respondents perceived themselves as physically very healthy and unrestricted in their work and daily activities.

5.3.4.5 Problems due to emotional health

This subsection reports three items assessing emotional health and wellness. Falun Gong respondents were asked to report if they had difficulty with their work or other daily activities due to emotional problems, such as feeling anxious and/or depressed. The majority of Falun Gong respondents (95%, n=341) indicated that they did not have to reduce time spent on work. Most Falun Gong respondents reported they did not do less than they liked and were able to perform their tasks carefully. Table 5.6 shows the frequency and percentage distribution for the three items on problems due to emotional health.

Table 5.6 Problems with work due to emotional health (Falun Gong respondents)

	Reduce Work Time		Do Less than You Like		Did Not Do Work as Carefully	
	F	%	F	%	F	%
No	341	94.7	313	86.9	333	92.5
Yes	15	4.2	42	11.7	21	5.8
Missing	4	1.1	5	1.4	6	1.7
Total	360	100.0	360	100.0	360	100.0

F=Frequency

5.3.4.6 Extent to which physical/emotional problems affect social activities

The Falun Gong respondents were provided with five options to report the extent to which physical and emotional problems had affected normal social activities with family, friends, neighbors, or other groups of individuals. As shown in Chart 5.19, the majority of Falun Gong respondents were "not at all" affected. No Falun Gong respondent reported being "extremely" affected by physical and emotional problems.

Chart 5.19 Extent to which physical/emotional problems affect social activities of Falun Gong respondents

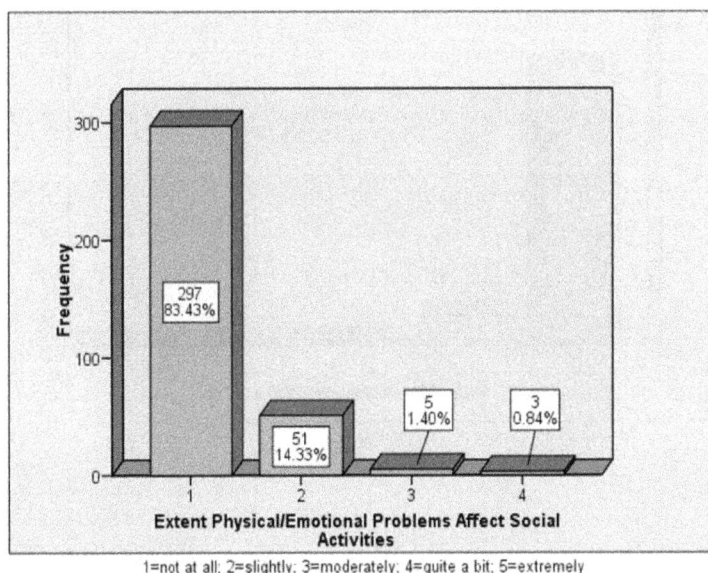

1=not at all; 2=slightly; 3=moderately; 4=quite a bit; 5=extremely

Note: Missing=4

5.3.4.7 Physical pain and how much pain had affected normal work

This subsection reports two items on physical pain and how much pain had affected normal work for Falun Gong respondents. Five options were provided to gauge how much physical or bodily pain they had during the four weeks prior to completing the survey. About two-thirds of Falun Gong respondents (67.7%, n=244) reported having no pain, while 24% (n=87) reported having "mild" pain. Two respondents reported having severe pain, while another three indicated having very severe pain during the past four weeks prior to completing survey.

The Falun Gong respondents were asked to report how much physical or bodily pain had affected their normal work at home and outside the home across five options as illustrated in Chart 5.20. The majority of Falun Gong respondents (88%, n=314, missing=5) reported "not at all." One respondent reported being extremely affected by pain.

Chart 5.20 Physical pain affecting normal work for Falun Gong respondents

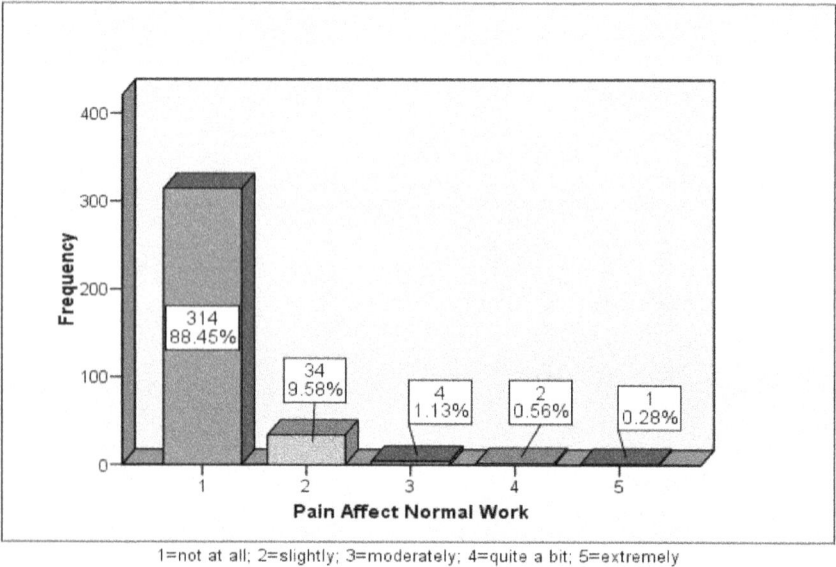

1=not at all; 2=slightly; 3=moderately; 4=quite a bit; 5=extremely

5.3.4.8 Feelings and how things had been

This subsection reports nine items from the SF-36 that measure vitality and mental health-wellness. Falun Gong respondents were provided with six options and asked to choose one that best described the way they felt and how things had been for them. Eighty-one percent of Falun Gong respondents (n=293) reported they were either full of life all or most of the time. A total of 83% of Falun Gong respondents (n=298) reported feeling calm and peaceful all or most of the time. Likewise, 82% of Falun Gong respondents (n=294) indicated having a lot of energy all or most of the time, while 84% (n=303) identified themselves as being a happy person all or most of the time. Less than five Falun Gong respondents reported "none of the time" for the four positive mental states. Table 5.7 and Table 5.9 show the frequency and percentage distribution for their positive feelings and healthy mental states, and negative feelings and unhealthy mental states respectively.

Table 5.7 Positive feelings and how things had been for Falun Gong respondents

Option	Full of Life F	Full of Life %	Calm & Peaceful F	Calm & Peaceful %	A Lot of Energy F	A Lot of Energy %	Been a Happy Person F	Been a Happy Person %
1	116	32.2	82	22.8	76	21.1	89	24.72
2	177	49.2	216	60.0	218	60.5	214	59.44
3	39	10.8	53	14.7	47	13.1	40	11.11
4	16	4.4	6	1.7	13	3.6	7	1.94
5	2	0.6	0	0	2	0.6	3	0.83
6	5	1.4	0	0	0	0	2	0.56
Missing	5	1.4	3	0.8	4	1.1	5	1.49
Total	360	100	360	100	360	100	360	100

1=All of the time; 2=Most of the time; 3=A good bit of the time; 4=Some of the time; 5=A little of the time; 6=None of the time. F=Frequency

As indicated in Table 5.8, the majority of Falun Gong respondents (86%, n=308) reported they were either not nervous or only "a little of the time." When asked if they felt "down in the dumps," 73% of Falun Gong respondents (n=262) stated "none of the time." One respondent indicated feeling blue, worn out or tired "all of the time" for each of these four items.

Table 5.8 Negative feelings and how things had been for Falun Gong respondents

Option	Very Nervous		Felt Down in the Dumps		Downhearted and blue		Worn out		Tired	
	F	%	F	%	F	%	F	%	F	%
1	202	56.1	262	72.8	204	56.7	165	45.8	70	19.4
2	106	29.4	75	20.8	126	35.0	147	40.8	209	58.1
3	39	10.8	12	3.3	19	5.3	29	8.1	61	16.9
4	5	1.4	2	0.6	5	1.4	10	2.7	12	3.3
5	3	0.8	3	0.8	2	0.6	2	0.6	3	0.8
6	2	0.6	2	0.6	1	0.3	1	0.3	1	0.3
Missing	3	0.8	4	1.1	3	0.8	6	1.7	4	1.1
Total	360	100	360	100	360	100	360	100	360	100

6=All of the time; 5=Most of the time; 4=A good bit of the time; 3=Some of the time; 2=A little of the time; 1=None of the time. F=Frequency

Overall, the majority of Falun Gong respondents perceived themselves as happy, calm, peaceful, feeling full of life, and having a lot of energy. Most of them reported they did not feel nervous, downhearted, blue or depressed, or worn out and tired.

5.3.4.9 Time physical/emotional problems affected social activities

The Falun Gong respondents were asked to indicate how much of the time physical or emotional problems had affected their social life. Eighty-one percent of respondents (n=292) indicated "none of the time," while 13% (n=48) reported "a little of the time" and 2.8% (n=10) rated "some of the time." Only 1.4% (n=5) reported that physical and emotional problems had interfered with social activities either most or all of the time.

5.3.4.10 Falun Gong respondents' perceptions of their health-wellness status

This subsection reports the last four items of the SF-36 assessing the general health-wellness status of respondents. Falun Gong respondents were asked for their perceptions and reports of their health, and to rate four statements, two in negative and two in positive terms, as shown in Table 5.9 and Table 5.10

respectively. The majority of Falun Gong respondents (87%, n=313) reported it was "definitely false" that they "seem to get sick a little easier than other people." Likewise the majority (90%, n=324) did not expect their health to get worse. When asked to rate their health-wellness status in positive terms, nearly two-thirds of Falun Gong respondents (65%, n=234) reported "I am as healthy as anybody I know" was definitely true, while over three-quarters (76%, n=274) perceived their health as excellent.

Table 5.9 displays the frequency and percentage distribution for Falun Gong respondents for the two negative statements, "I seem to get sick a little easier than other people," and "I expect my health to get worse."

Table 5.9 Falun Gong respondents' perceptions of their health-wellness status from two negative statements

Option		I seem to get sick a little easier		I expect my health to get worse	
		Frequency	Percent	Frequency	Percent
1	Definitely false	313	86.9	324	90
2	Mostly false	22	6.1	24	6.7
3	Don't know	13	3.6	7	1.9
4	Mostly true	1	0.3	0	0
5	Definitely true	4	1.1	1	0.3
Sub-Total		353	98.0	356	98.9
Missing		7	1.9	4	1.1
Total		360	100	360	100

Table 5.10 displays the frequency and percentage distribution for two positive statements, "I am as healthy as anybody I know," and "My health is excellent."

Table 5.10 Falun Gong respondents' perceptions of their health-wellness status from two positive statements

Option		I am as healthy as anybody I know		My health is excellent	
		Frequency	Percent	Frequency	Percent
1	Definitely true	234	65.0	274	76.11
2	Mostly true	69	19.2	75	20.83
3	Don't know	27	7.5	3	0.83
4	Mostly false	12	3.3	4	1.11
5	Definitely false	13	3.6	1	0.28
Sub-Total		355	98.6	357	99.17
Missing		5	1.4	3	0.83
Total		360	100.0	360	100.0

Findings from the SF-36 items showed Falun Gong respondents perceived themselves as physically, mentally, and emotionally very healthy. The majority reported an optimistic and positive outlook of their own health status.

This concludes the data reporting for Falun Gong respondents.

CHAPTER 6

Findings for Non–Falun Gong Respondents

6.1 Chapter overview

This chapter presents the findings for non–Falun Gong respondents. The findings are presented in three sections. The first comprises the demographic profile, and the second the medical history and health status of the non–Falun Gong respondents. The third section presents the findings from the Short Form (SF-36) Health Survey.

6.2 Section 1: Demographic profile

Section 1 reports the demographic profile of 230 non–Falun Gong respondents. Overall, like the Falun Gong group, there were more female non–Falun Gong respondents. Nearly 50% of non–Falun Gong respondents were married, had tertiary education qualifications, and came from diverse ethnic backgrounds. Non–Falun Gong respondents were more likely to have English as their first language and mainly resided in Australia and New Zealand or Canada and the United States. Comparison data between Falun Gong and non–Falun Gong respondents is summarized in Chapter 8. All data was reported and analyzed using descriptive statistics and presented according to the order of the items in the HW2 (see Appendix 4).

6.2.1 Gender distribution

There were more female than male non–Falun Gong respondents as shown in Chart 6.1.

Chart 6.1 Gender distribution

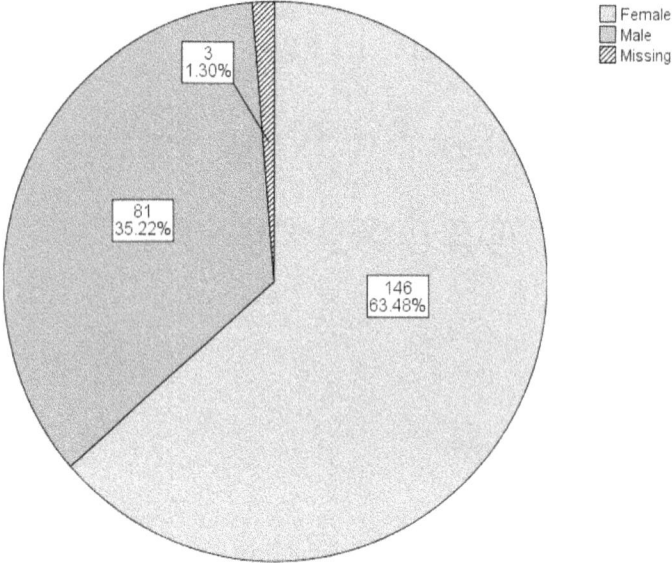

6.2.2 Age range

The non–Falun Gong respondents were asked to identify their age range. Similar to the Falun Gong group, the average age of non–Falun Gong respondents fell between the 30 to 39 years and 40 to 49 years of age range, as shown in Chart 6.2.

6.2.3 Relationship status

Nearly half of non–Falun Gong respondents (48%, n=110, missing=2) were married as shown in Chart 6.3. There were 19 non–Falun Gong respondents in de facto relationships, as opposed to five cases for Falun Gong respondents.

Chart 6.2 Age range of non–Falun Gong respondents

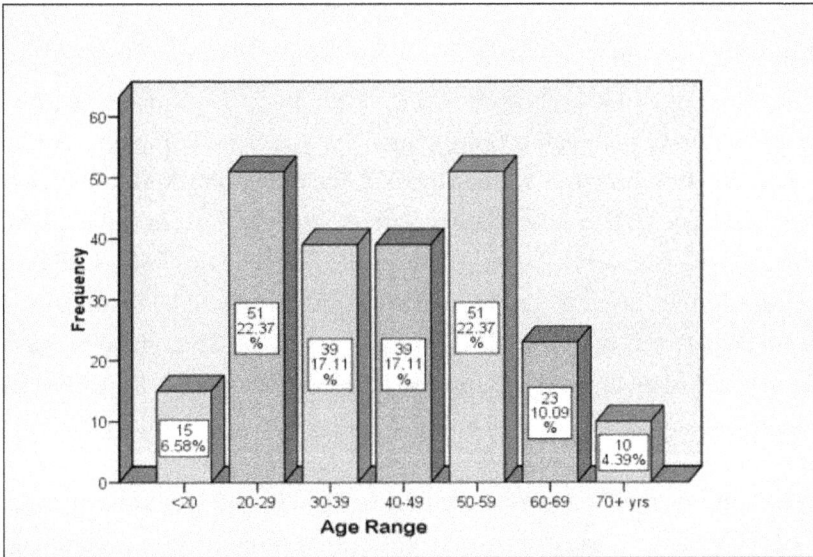

Note: Missing=2

Chart 6.3 Relationship status of non–Falun Gong respondents

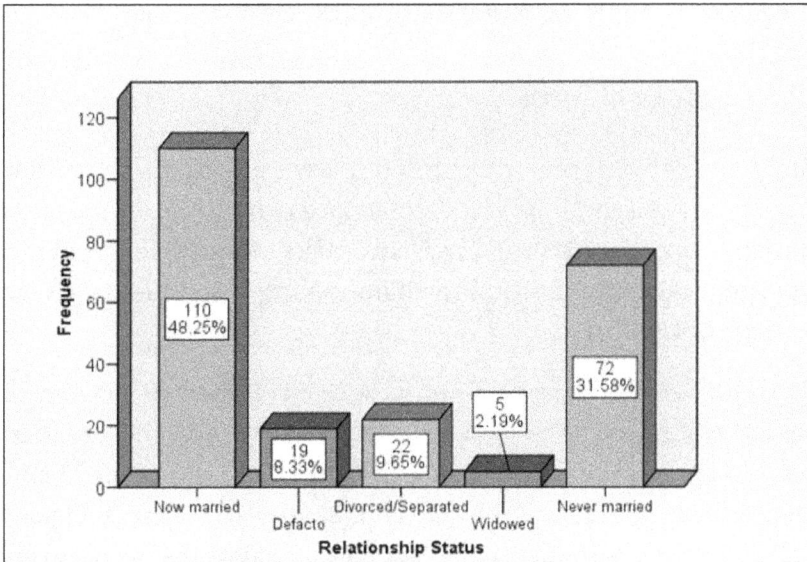

6.2.4 Ethnicity

No prescriptive range of ethnicity was provided, with non–Falun Gong respondents free to identify their ethnic origin. Like the Falun Gong group, the ethnicities of non–Falun Gong respondents were wide-ranging. A total of 33 different ethnicities were identified, including one Arab, Australian Aborigine, Australian Jew, Maori, Native North American Indian, New Zealand Cook Islander, Lebanese/Polynesian, Persian, two Burmese, Polish, Russians; three Filipinos, and five Africans. Others identified themselves as Anglo-Celtic, Acadian Cuban, Caucasian, Indian, Italian, Greek, Irish, Scottish, Spanish, Sri Lankan, Welsh, Japanese, Korean, Malaysian, Singaporean, Indonesian, and Thai.

Several non–Falun Gong respondents described themselves as having dual ethnic origins, such as African-Indian, Eurasians, Indo-Chinese, Chinger-Burmese and Italian-Greek. Individuals of Chinese ethnicity comprised the largest group (27.4%, n=63). Eighteen percent of non–Falun Gong respondents (n=42) identified themselves as Caucasians, 23% (n=52) identified themselves as Australians, while others as Americans (n=5) and Canadians (n=2). Due to the ethnic diversity, it was unrealistic to display the data visually.

6.2.5 Country of birth

The non–Falun Gong respondents were asked to state their country of birth. The researcher classified the nominated countries for country of birth and also country of residence consistent with the method for Falun Gong respondents. (Refer to Section 5.3.1.5.)

A total of 37 different countries of birth were identified. Those born in Australia and New Zealand comprised the largest category (40%, n=92, missing=3), and those born in Asia the second highest category (21%, n=48). Only 23 non–Falun Gong respondents (10%) were born in mainland China, as opposed to 97 Falun Gong respondents (27%). Chart 6.4 shows the frequency and percentage distribution for country of birth of non–Falun Gong respondents.

Chart 6.4 Country of birth of non–Falun Gong respondents

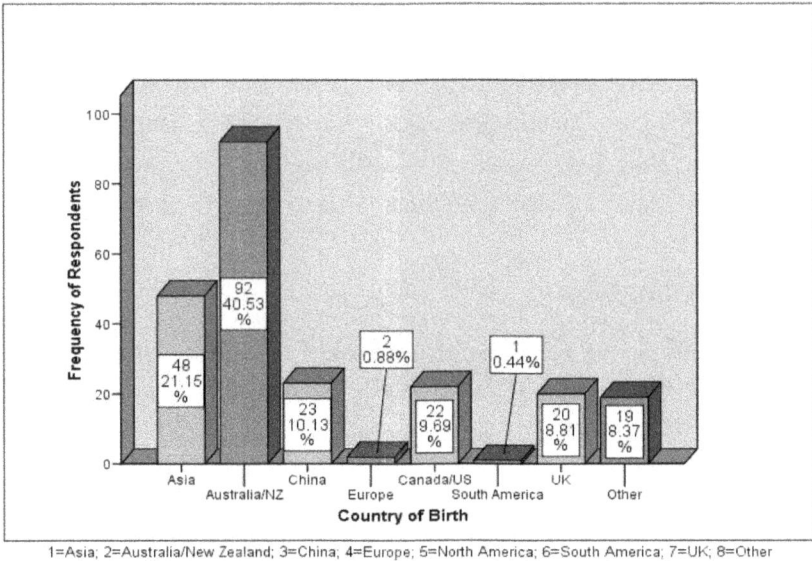

1=Asia; 2=Australia/New Zealand; 3=China; 4=Europe; 5=North America; 6=South America; 7=UK; 8=Other

Chart 6.5 Country of residence of non–Falun Gong respondents

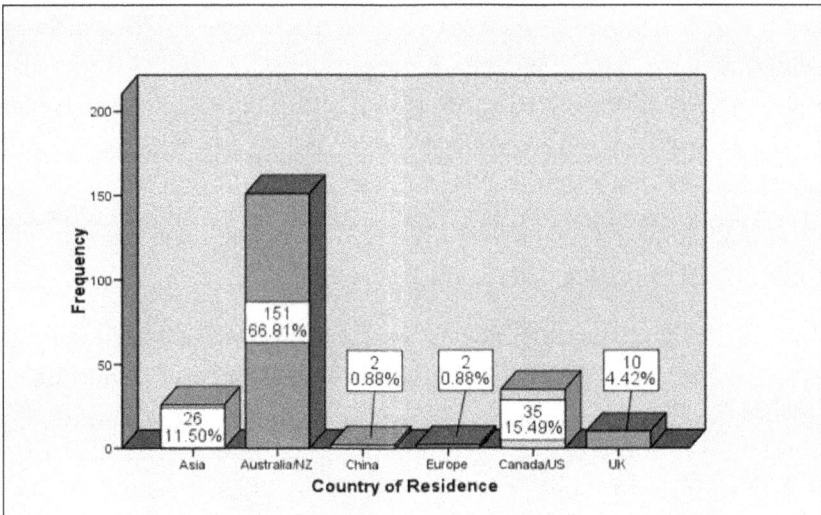

6.2.6 Country of residence

The non–Falun Gong respondents were asked to specify their country of residence. The countries identified were classified as for country of birth. Like Falun Gong respondents, the majority of non–Falun Gong respondents (82%, n=186, missing=4) resided in two main regions of the world: Australia and New Zealand; and Canada and the U.S., as shown in Chart 6.5.

6.2.7 First language

The non–Falun Gong respondents were asked to indicate whether or not English was their first language. Compared to Falun Gong respondents, there were more non–Falun Gong respondents (57%, n=130) who reported English as their first language, while 41% (n=94) indicated the reverse. The diversity of non–Falun Gong respondents' ethnicities were reflected in the variety of languages they spoke that were not English. Fifty-three non–Falun Gong respondents (23%) reported their first language as either Mandarin or Cantonese, or other Chinese dialects such as Hokkien. Non–Falun Gong respondents came from diverse ethnic backgrounds and reported different first languages, ranging from Arabic, Farsi Iranian, and South African Sotho to a variety of Asian, European, and Eastern European languages. These included Bahasa Indonesia, Bahasa Malaysia, Burmese, Dhivehi Fijian language, Fijian Hindi, Indian Malayalam, Japanese, Korean, Tagalog, Tamil, Thai, Dutch, Hungarian, Italian, Lithuanian, Greek, Polish, Portuguese, Russian, Spanish, and Turkish.

6.2.8 Highest education level

Most non–Falun Gong respondents were tertiary educated, like the Falun Gong group. Over 50% of non–Falun Gong respondents (n=115, missing=6) reported having university degree qualifications, as shown in Chart 6.6.

Chart 6.6 Highest education level of non–Falun Gong respondents

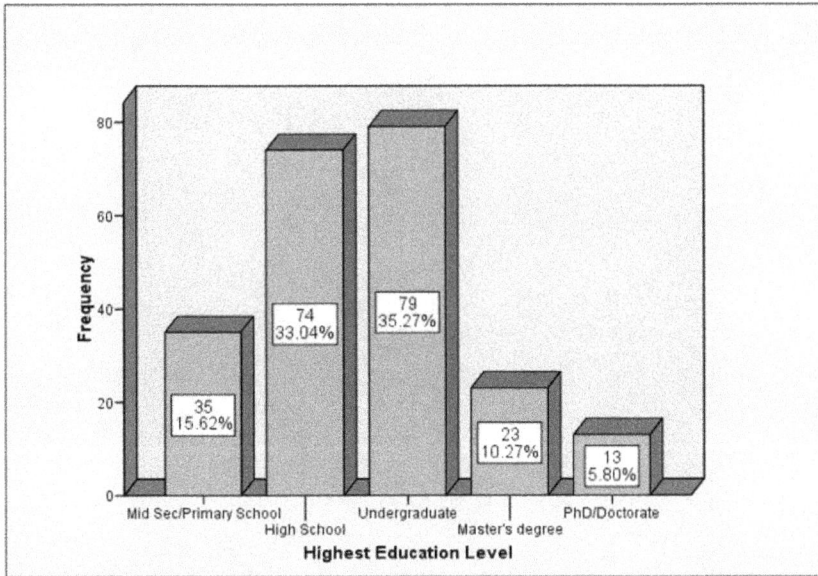

6.2.9 Occupations

Consistent with Falun Gong respondents, ANZSCO (Australian Bureau of Statistics & Statistics New Zealand, 2006) was used as a guide to categorize the responses of the non–Falun Gong respondents. See Appendix 5, which details the major categories and subcategories of occupations as derived from the ABS (2006) and SNZ (2006). Non–Falun Gong respondents were also from diverse occupational backgrounds, ranging from unemployment, being students, skilled and unskilled labor jobs to professional, executive, and senior administrative positions. Business/computer information technology professionals comprised the largest number of non–Falun Gong respondents (16.2%, n=36), clerical, sales, administrative and service workers the second largest category (14.9%, n=33), while those retired/performing home duties, and students were third and fourth respectively. Skilled and unskilled laborers and the unemployed formed the smallest occupational categories of 2.7% for non–Falun Gong respondents (n=6). Chart 6.7 shows the frequency and percentage distribution across the major categories of occupations of non–Falun Gong respondents.

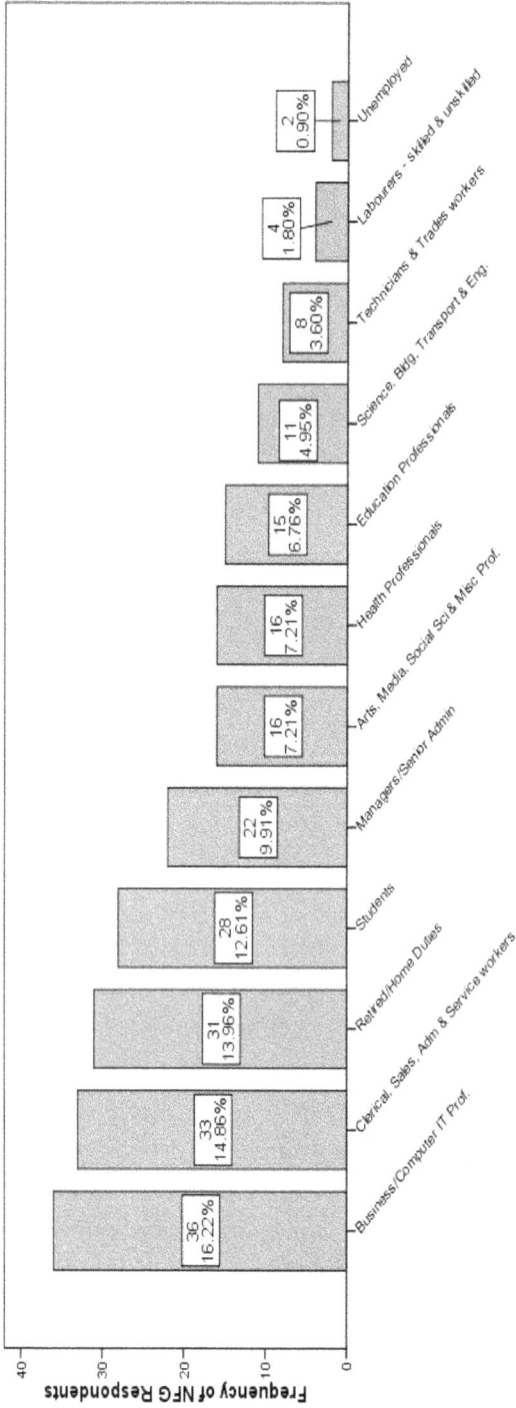

Chart 6.7 Occupations of non-Falun Gong respondents

Note: Missing = 8

6.3 Section 2: Medical history and health status

Section 2 comprised 13 items seeking self-reports from non–Falun Gong respondents about their medical history, number of medical consultations, reasons for medical consultations, medication intake history, medical and health expenses, cigarette smoking, alcohol consumption, and recreational drug use habits. Overall, non–Falun Gong respondents were healthy and led a moderate lifestyle. They visited medical practitioners more frequently, took more medications and health supplements, and spent more on medical and health expenses than Falun Gong respondents. They were typically non-smokers, who consumed alcohol, and the few who reported taking recreational drugs had no intention of stopping or changing their lifestyle.

6.3.1 Visits to medical practitioners

The non–Falun Gong respondents were asked to state the number of visits they made to a medical practitioner during the past six months. More than half of non–Falun Gong respondents (56%, n=127, missing=4) consulted a medical practitioner at least one to three times. Chart 6.8 shows the frequency and percentage distribution for the number of visits to a medical practitioner by non–Falun Gong respondents.

Chart 6.8 Number of visits to medical practitioners

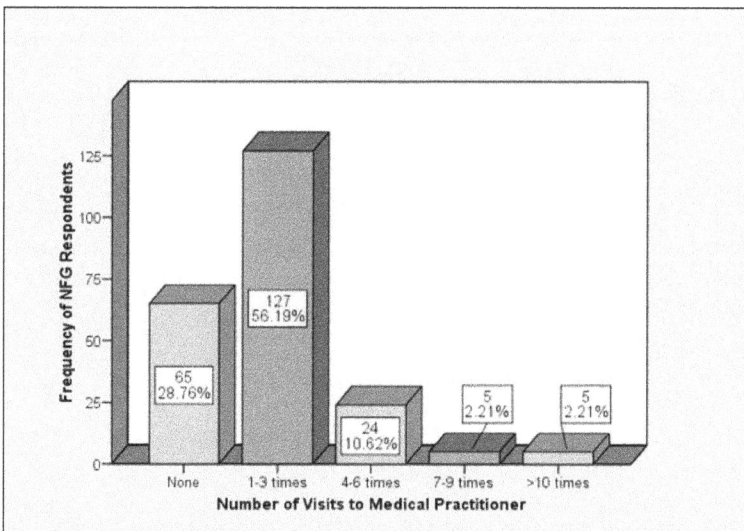

6.3.2 Reason for medical visits

The qualitative data for Item 13 is reported in Chapter 7.

6.3.3 Use of medication and health supplements

The non–Falun Gong respondents were provided with a range of medication and health supplement options and asked to identify all that applied to their situation. Sixty-five percent of non–Falun Gong respondents (n=141) reported using a variety of combinations of prescription and over the counter drugs, Chinese and Western herbal remedies, homeopathic remedies, and vitamins and health supplements. Two non–Falun Gong respondents reported using all the seven options.

Table 6.1 shows the frequency and percentage distributions in the use of each of the different types of medication and supplements by non–Falun Gong respondents.

Table 6.1 Use of medications and health supplements by non–Falun Gong respondents

Options	Description of Items	F*	Percent*
1	None	81	35.2
2	Prescription drugs (medical)	74	32.1
3	Over counter drugs, e.g. Panadol, Aspirin	38	16.5
4	Chinese herbal remedies	13	5.6
5	Western herbal remedies	7	3.0
6	Homeopathic remedies	9	3.9
7	Vitamins and health supplements	66	28.6
Missing		8	3.5

* The frequency and percentage distribution show the number of times each option was selected, and hence do not add up to the total number of non–Falun Gong respondents (n=230) or to 100%.

6.3.4 Medical and health expenses

The non–Falun Gong respondents were asked to report all their medical and health expenses, which included prescriptions, herbal remedies, supplements, naturopathic consultations, vitamins and health supplements during the past six months. Two-thirds of non–Falun Gong respondents (67%, n=153) reported spending money on medical and health expenses. They were asked to provide the total amount spent in their local currency with the intention of converting all the reported expenses to Australian dollars. However, currency conversion to the Australian dollar made it impossible to draw any conclusions or comparisons because of the vast differences in the standards and costs of living in different countries. Hence, it was decided not to report this item in any visual form.

6.3.5 Cigarette smoking, alcohol intake and recreational drug use

The non–Falun Gong respondents were asked to report whether or not they were involved in substance use, such as cigarette smoking, alcohol consumption and recreational drug use. They were asked to state the amount used and if they had plans to stop. Non–Falun Gong respondents were generally non-smokers and consumed alcohol. Those who reported consuming alcohol and taking recreational drugs had no plans to stop.

6.3.5.1 Cigarette smoking

Chart 6.9 shows the percentage and frequency distribution of cigarette smoking by non–Falun Gong respondents. Those who smoked cigarettes reported less than 10 to 20 cigarettes per day and 63% of them (n=20) planned to quit smoking.

Chart 6.9 Cigarette smoking by non–Falun Gong respondents

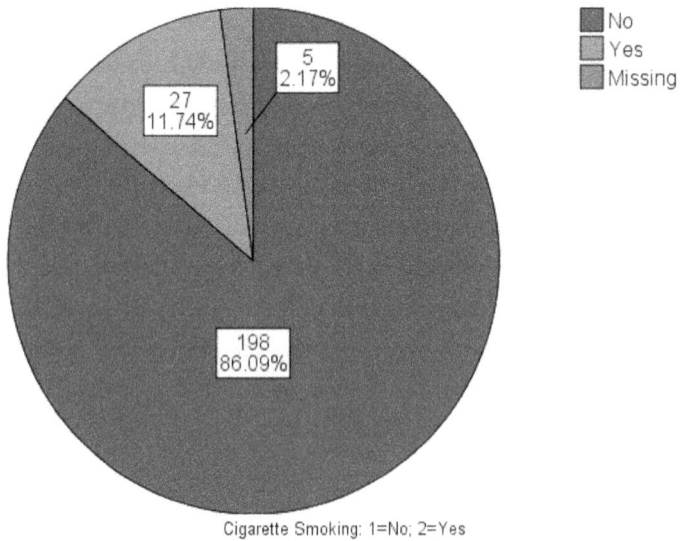

No
Yes
Missing

5
2.17%

27
11.74%

198
86.09%

Cigarette Smoking: 1=No; 2=Yes

6.3.5.2 Alcohol consumption

About two-thirds of non–Falun Gong respondents (60%, n=138) consumed alcohol, as shown in Chart 6.10.

Chart 6.10 Alcohol consumption by non–Falun Gong respondents

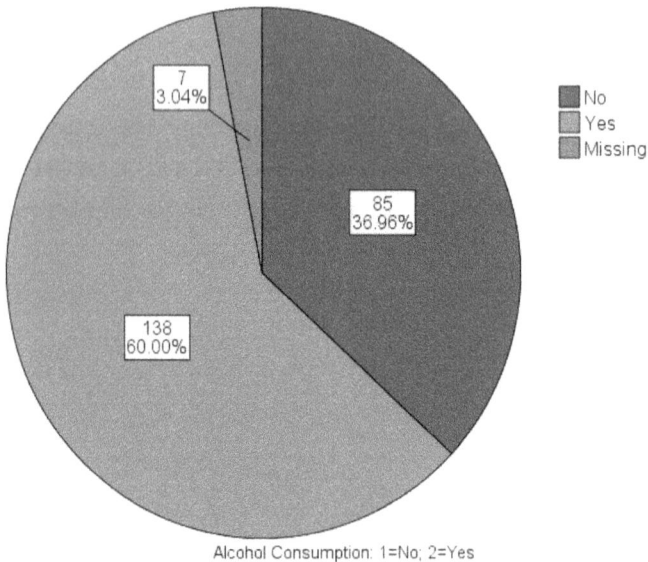

No
Yes
Missing

7
3.04%

85
36.96%

138
60.00%

Alcohol Consumption: 1=No; 2=Yes

The quantity of alcohol intake reported varied from one glass to 200ml of wine a week, 750ml of wine per day, or 375ml to 1,500ml of beer per day. Due to the varied responses, it is problematical to derive any conclusions from the data on the amount of alcohol consumed per day by non–Falun Gong respondents and this has not been displayed. When asked in a separate question (Item 21), 52% of non–Falun Gong respondents (n=119) reported having no plans to stop alcohol consumption.

6.3.5.3 Recreational drug use

The majority of non–Falun Gong respondents (92%, n=211) reported not taking any recreational drugs, as shown in Chart 6.11. Of the eight non–Falun Gong respondents who did report taking recreational drugs: one took ecstasy; two respondents used marijuana; and one respondent indicated a mixture of marijuana, ecstasy, as well as other drugs. Those who reported using recreational drugs stated they had no plans to stop.

Chart 6.11 Recreational drug use by non–Falun Gong respondents

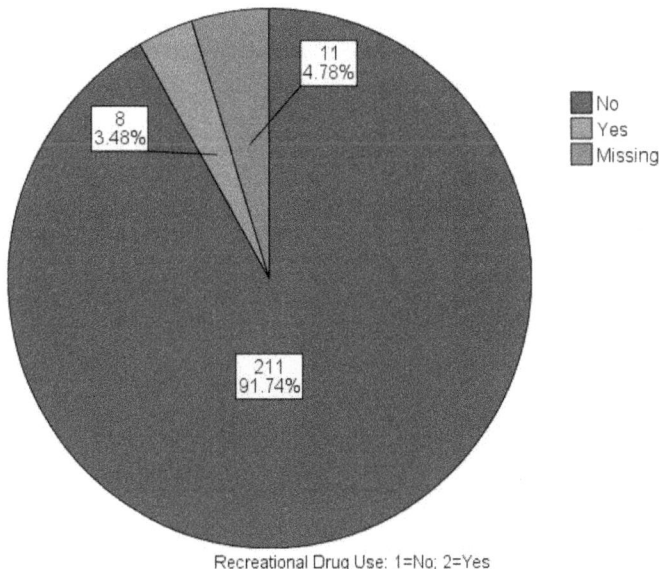

Recreational Drug Use: 1=No; 2=Yes

6.4 Section 3: Short Form Health Survey (SF-36)

Section 3 of HW2 reported data from the SF-36, which comprised 36 items seeking self-reports from non–Falun Gong respondents about their general, physical, mental, and emotional health status, how they felt and how well they were able to perform their normal daily activities. (See Appendix 4 for the HW2.)

Overall, non–Falun Gong respondents perceived themselves as healthy individuals; 41% of them (n=95) reported "very good" general health status and another 31% (n=72) reported "good" health status. Four non–Falun Gong respondents (1.7%) perceived their health status to be "poor." While most non–Falun Gong respondents were not limited by poor health in their normal daily activities, many reported some degree of limitation for vigorous activities, such as running, lifting heavy objects, participating in strenuous sports, or climbing several flights of stairs.

6.4.1 General health status

The non–Falun Gong respondents were asked to indicate their general health status according to a range of five options, as shown in Chart 6.12.

Chart 6.12 General health status of non–Falun Gong respondents

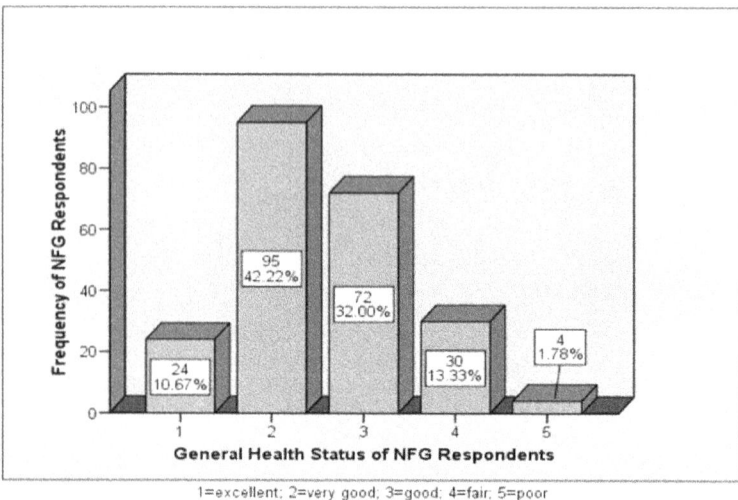

1=excellent; 2=very good; 3=good; 4=fair; 5=poor

Note: Missing=5

Most non–Falun Gong respondents either reported their general health status as very good or good, whereas most Falun Gong respondents reported excellent to very good health status.

6.4.2 General health a year ago

The non–Falun Gong respondents were provided with five options (see Appendix 4 for HW2 Survey) to indicate their general health as compared to one year ago. Ten percent of non–Falun Gong respondents (n=23) rated their general health as "much better" than a year ago. Nearly 20% of non–Falun Gong respondents (n= 45) reported being "somewhat better," while 10% (n=23) reported experiencing deterioration in their general health.

6.4.3 How health limits daily activities

This subsection reports 10 items from the SF-36 relating to the assessment of physical health. Non–Falun Gong respondents were provided with three options to indicate whether their health had limited them from a range of daily activities that they might do during a typical day. Apart from vigorous activities, most non–Falun Gong respondents reported that their health had not limited them from performing their daily activities. More than half of non–Falun Gong respondents (55%, n=127) reported their health had limited them in doing vigorous activities, while 41% (n=94) stated they were not limited at all. Thirty-eight percent (n=88) reported their health had limited them in climbing several flights of stairs, while 58% (n=133) were not limited at all.

About two-thirds of non–Falun Gong respondents reported not being limited by their health with moderate activities, like moving a small table or using a domestic vacuum cleaner, bending, kneeling, or walking more than a mile, as shown in Table 6.2. Nearly 75% of non–Falun Gong respondents reported not being limited at all by their health to perform daily tasks, such as carrying groceries, climbing one flight of stairs, or walking several blocks.

Table 6.2 displays the frequency and percentage distribution of non–Falun Gong respondents for the 10 items relating to physical health.

Table 6.2 How health limits daily activities of non–Falun Gong respondents

	Vigorous Activities		Moderate Activities		Lift/Carry Groceries		Climb Several Stairs		Climb One Flight of Stairs		Bend, Kneel or Stoop		Walk More than a Mile		Walk Several Blocks		Walk One Block		Bathe or Dress yourself	
	F	%	F	%	F	%	F	%	F	%	F	%	F	%	F	%	F	%	F	%
1	94	40.9	157	68.3	169	73.5	133	57.8	176	76.5	150	65.2	157	68.3	173	75.2	189	82.1	200	87.0
2	93	40.4	50	21.7	37	16.1	61	26.5	29	12.6	51	22.2	42	18.3	29	12.6	16	7.0	6	2.6
3	34	14.8	16	7.0	16	7.0	27	11.7	17	7.4	19	8.3	22	9.6	19	8.3	17	7.4	17	7.4
Sub-Total	221	96.1	223	97.0	222	96.5	221	96.1	222	96.5	220	95.7	221	96.1	221	96.1	222	96.5	223	97.0
M	9	3.9	7	3.0	8	3.5	9	3.9	8	3.5	10	4.3	9	3.9	9	3.9	8	3.5	7	3.0
Total	230	100	230	100	230	100	230	100	230	100	230	100	230	100	230	100	230	100	230	100

For visual clarity, gridlines are added.

Overall, other than vigorous activities, most non–Falun Gong respondents perceived themselves as physically healthy and not limited from doing moderate daily activities. Their self-perceived reports of physical health limitations were not as positive and optimistic as Falun Gong respondents. See Chapter 8 for the tabulated highlights of differences between Falun Gong and non–Falun Gong respondents for these items.

6.4.4 Problems due to physical health

This subsection reports four items from the SF-36 assessing physical health-wellness. Non–Falun Gong respondents were asked to indicate if they had any problems with their work or other regular daily activities due to their physical health. Table 6.3 displays the frequency (F) and percentage distribution of non–Falun Gong respondents for the four items.

Table 6.3 Problems with work due to physical health for four items

	Reduce Work Time		Do Less than You Like		Limited in Work or Activities		Difficulty Doing Work	
	F	%	F	%	F	%	F	%
No	194	84.3	167	72.6	182	79.1	185	80.4
Yes	31	13.5	57	24.8	40	17.4	38	16.5
Missing	5	2.2	6	2.6	8	3.5	7	3.0
Total	230	100.0	230	100.0	230	100.0	230	100.0

F=Frequency

Overall, non–Falun Gong respondents reported not having a lot of problems with their work and daily activities due to physical health. The majority reported they did not have to reduce work time, do less than they like, or feel limited in the kind of work they could perform, or had any difficulty doing their tasks and other activities.

6.4.5 Problems with work due to emotional health

This subsection reports three items from the SF-36 assessing emotional health-wellness. Non–Falun Gong respondents were asked to indicate if they had difficulty with their work or other regular daily activities due to emotional problems, such as feeling anxious or depressed. Over three-quarters of non–Falun Gong respondents reported they did not have to reduce work time and were able to do their work, as carefully as usual, while 70% (n=160) reported that they did not have to do less than they like. Table 6.4 displays the frequency (F) and percentage distribution of non–Falun Gong respondents for these three items.

Table 6.4 Problems with work due to emotional health for three items

| | Reduce Work Time | | Do Less than You Like | | Did Not Do Work as Carefully as Usual | |
	F	%	F	%	F	%
No	181	78.7	160	69.6	183	79.6
Yes	43	18.7	63	27.4	41	17.8
Missing	6	2.6	7	3.0	6	2.6
Total	230	100.0	230	100.0	230	100.0

F=Frequency

6.4.6 Extent to which physical/emotional problems affect social activities

The non–Falun Gong respondents were asked to indicate the extent to which physical and emotional problems had affected normal social activities with family, friends, neighbors, or other groups of individuals. None of the non–Falun Gong respondents reported being "extremely" affected by physical and emotional problems, while four percent (n=10, missing=5) reported being affected "quite a bit." Chart 6.13 displays the frequency and percentage distribution of physical and emotional problems affecting social activities of non–Falun Gong respondents.

Chart 6.13 Extent to which physical/emotional problems affect social activities of non–Falun Gong respondents

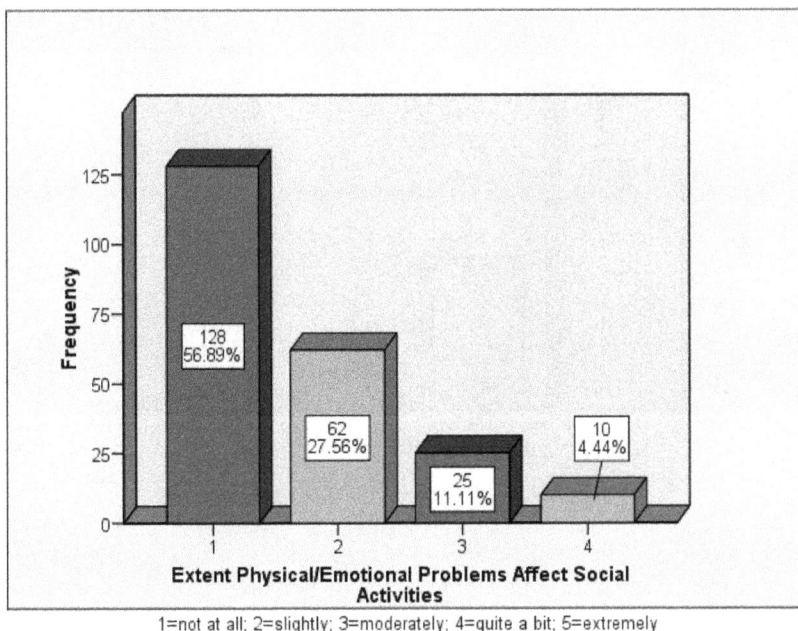

1=not at all; 2=slightly; 3=moderately; 4=quite a bit; 5=extremely

6.4.7 Physical pain and how much pain had affected normal work

This subsection reports two items on physical pain and how much pain had affected normal work. Non–Falun Gong respondents were given five options and asked to gauge how much physical or bodily pain they had during the four weeks prior to completing the survey. Forty-five percent of non–Falun Gong respondents (n=103) reported having no pain, while 50% (n=115) reported mild to moderate pain.

Non–Falun Gong respondents were also asked to indicate how much pain had affected normal work at home and outside the home. Nearly two-thirds of non–Falun Gong respondents (63%, n=142, missing=6) reported not being affected, as shown in Chart 6.14.

Chart 6.14 Physical pain affecting normal work

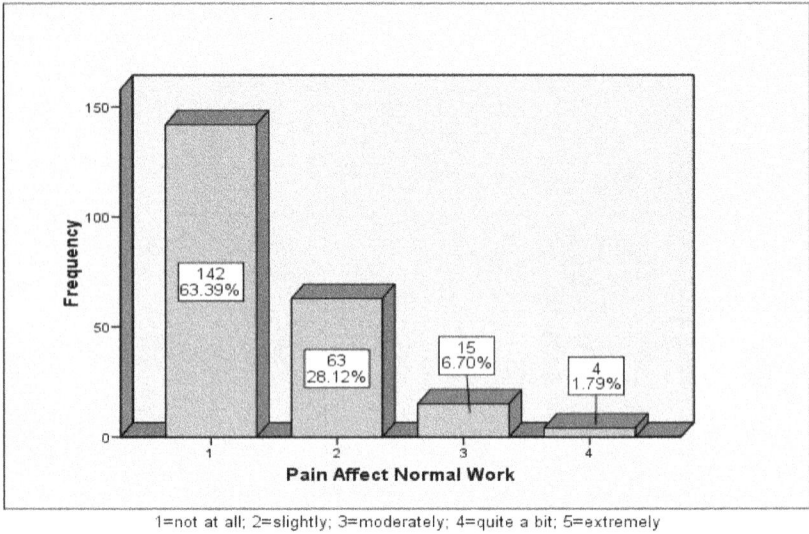

1=not at all; 2=slightly; 3=moderately; 4=quite a bit; 5=extremely

6.4.8 Feelings and how things had been

This section reports nine items from the SF-36 that measure vitality and mental health-wellness. Non–Falun Gong respondents were given six options and asked to choose one that best described how they felt and how things had been for them. A lower scale rating indicated a positive health outcome, while a higher scale indicated a poor health outcome.

Table 6.5 shows the frequency and percentage distribution of non–Falun Gong respondents for their positive feelings and healthy mental states. Fifty-five percent of non–Falun Gong respondents (n=127) reported they were either full of life all or most of the time. About two-thirds of non-Falun Gong respondents (n=147) indicated being a happy person, all or most of the time, as shown in Table 6.5.

Table 6.5 Positive feelings and how things had been

No	Full of Life		Calm & Peaceful		A Lot of Energy		Been a Happy Person	
	F	%	F	%	F	%	F	%
1	23	10.0	12	5.2	11	4.8	28	12.2
2	104	45.2	90	39.1	89	38.7	119	51.7
3	40	17.4	52	22.6	48	20.9	41	17.8
4	43	18.7	40	17.4	50	21.7	24	10.4
5	11	4.8	20	8.7	18	7.8	10	4.3
6	2	0.9	7	3.0	8	3.5	2	0.9
Missing	7	3.0	9	3.9	6	2.6	6	2.6
Total	230	100.0	230	100.0	230	100.0	230	100.0

1=All of the time; 2=Most of the time; 3=A good bit of the time; 4=Some of the time; 5=A little of the time; 6=None of the time. F=Frequency

Table 6.6 shows the frequency and percentage distribution of non–Falun Gong respondents for their negative feelings and unhealthy mental states. About one-third of non–Falun Gong respondents reported not feeling nervous (34%, n=77) or downhearted and blue (33%, n=76), while nearly half (49%, n=113) indicated not feeling "down in the dumps."

Table 6.6 Negative feelings and how things had been

No	Very Nervous		Felt Down in the Dumps		Downhearted and blue		Worn out		Tired	
	F	%	F	%	F	%	F	%	F	%
1	77	33.5	113	49.1	76	33.0	24	10.4	10	4.4
2	85	38	71	30.9	83	36.1	74	32.2	79	34.4
3	36	15.8	26	11.3	48	20.9	77	33.5	77	33.5
4	12	5.2	9	3.9	13	5.7	33	14.3	25	10.9
5	9	3.9	4	1.7	3	1.3	12	5.2	25	10.9
6	3	1.3	0	0	1	0.4	2	0.9	7	3.0
Missing	8	3.5	7	3.0	6	2.6	8	3.5	7	3.0
Total	230	100.0	230	100.0	230	100.0	230	100.0	230	100.0

1=None of the time; 2=A little of the time; 3=Some of the time; 4=A good bit of the time; 5=Most of the time; 6=All of the time. F=Frequency

Overall, non–Falun Gong respondents perceived themselves as being happy, calm, peaceful, full of life, and having a lot of energy "most of the time." Few respondents reported feeling nervous, downhearted and blue, or worn out, while 11% (n=25) reported feeling tired "most of the time."

6.4.9 Time physical/emotional problems affected social activities

The non–Falun Gong respondents were given five options and asked to report how much of the time physical or emotional problems had affected their social activities, such as visiting friends and relatives. Over half of non–Falun Gong respondents (51%, n=118) indicated "none of the time," while the remaining 47% (n=107) reported being affected to varying extents of the time. About a quarter (26%, n=59) reported "a little of the time," 16% (n=36) "some of the time," while five percent (n=12) indicated being affected by physical and emotional problems all or most of the time.

6.4.10 Non–Falun Gong respondents' perceptions of their health-wellness status

This subsection reports the last four items of the SF-36 assessing general health-wellness. Non–Falun Gong respondents were asked for their perceptions and self-reports of their health and to rate four statements about their health, two in negative and two in positive terms, as shown in Table 6.7 and Table 6.8 respectively. Both tables display the frequency and percentage distribution for the two negative statements and the two positive statements respectively.

Nearly half of the non–Falun Gong respondents (47%, n=108) stated it was "definitely false" that they "seem to get sick a little easier than other people," while about a third (36.5%, n=84) indicated the same response when asked if they expect their health to get worse.

Table 6.7 Non–Falun Gong respondents' perceptions of their health-wellness status from two negative statements

		I seem to get sick a little easier		I expect my health to get worse	
Options		Frequency	Percent	Frequency	Percent
1	Definitely false	108	47.0	84	36.5
2	Mostly false	60	26.1	47	20.4
3	Don't know	35	15.2	76	33
4	Mostly true	18	7.8	11	4.8
5	Definitely true	4	1.7	6	2.6
Sub-Total		225	97.8	224	97.4
Missing		5	2.2	6	2.6
Total		230	100.0	230	100.0

When asked to rate their health in positive terms, less than a third of non–Falun Gong respondents (31%, n=72) reported it was "definitely true" that they were as healthy as anybody they knew, as indciated in Table 6.8. Only 19% of non–Falun Gong respondents (n=44) stated "definitely true" for the statement, "My health is excellent."

Table 6.8 Non–Falun Gong respondents' perceptions of their health-wellness status from two positive statements

		I am as healthy as anybody I know		My health is excellent	
Option		Frequency	Percent	Frequency	Percent
1	Definitely true	72	31.3	44	19.1
2	Mostly true	97	42.2	123	53.5
3	Don't know	32	13.9	25	10.9
4	Mostly false	18	7.8	25	10.9
5	Definitely false	5	2.2	8	3.5
Sub-Total		224	97.4	225	97.8
Missing		6	2.6	5	2.2
Total		230	100.0	230	100.0

Overall, Falun Gong respondents perceived themselves as physically, mentally, and emotionally very healthy, with most of them reporting an excellent general health status. Non–Falun Gong respondents also perceived themselves as healthy individuals, with many reporting very good general health status, but they tended not to be as positive and optimistic in their outlook and expectations about their general health status compared to Falun Gong respondents.

This concludes the quantitative data reporting for this research.

CHAPTER 7

Written Comments

7.1 Chapter overview

This chapter reports the qualitative data, which augments the scope and depth of the quantitative data findings (Hanson et al., 2005; Miles & Huberman, 1994; Sandelowski, 2000). Written responses were analyzed and interpreted separately following a simple three-level categorizing or clustering procedure adapted from approaches to qualitative content analysis, as discussed and used by writers and other health researchers (Graneheim & Lundman, 2004; Hanson et al., 2005; Miles & Huberman, 1994; Sharif & Masoumi, 2005).

The first level of analysis involved collating, describing and summarizing all the written responses into meaning units, while level two involved clustering these meaning units together into broad and similar categories (Graneheim & Lundman, 2004; Hanson et al., 2005; Sharif & Masoumi, 2005). For example, wisdom teeth, tooth extraction, broken tooth, teeth cleaning, and dental scaling were categorized as dental care, while muscularskeletal conditions included muscle pain, knee problem, shoulder and neck strain, ankle sprain, and so forth. The qualitative content was then transformed into quantified or numeric categories in the third level to obtain the frequency and percentage distribution for visual data presentation.

Table 7.1 shows examples of the three levels of categorizing of respondents' comments from Item 13 in Section 2 of HW1 and HW2.

Table 7.1 Examples of levels of categorizing - reasons for medical visit

Level 1: Meaning units	Level 2: Categories	Level 3: Quantified categories
A few stitches	Minor accidents	7=Other
Asthma	Chronic	4=Chronic/long-term
Broken tooth	Dental care	7=Other
General: Checkup	Medical checkup	2=Routine medical checkup
Colds	Minor viral infections	3=Minor health issues
Knee problem	Muscularskeletal	3=Minor health issues
Ovarian cancer	Life-threatening	6=Life-threatening
Teeth cleaning	Dental care	7=Other

Raw data for Item 13 indicated a total of 37 Falun Gong respondents and 156 non–Falun Gong respondents reporting one or multiple medical conditions as their reasons for visiting a medical practitioner. Each medical condition was first listed as a single meaning unit in Level 1, categorized in Level 2, and then transformed into quantified or numeric categories in Level 3, as shown in Table 7.2.

7.2 Written comments from Falun Gong respondents

This subsection reports the qualitative data in Section 2 and Section 3 of HW1 for Falun Gong respondents. Respondents' comments provided insight and an extra dimension to the overall findings from this research.

7.2.1 Item 13: Reason for medical visits by Falun Gong respondents

The Falun Gong respondents were asked to state the main reason(s) for consulting a medical practitioner. Their written responses were analyzed into seven categories as shown in Table 7.2. Where there were two or more listed medical conditions from the same respondent, these were categorized according to the most severe medical condition.

Table 7.2 Reasons for medical visits by Falun Gong respondents

Level	Category	Frequency	Percent
1	None/Not applicable	320	88.89
2	Routine medical checkup	2	0.56
3	Minor health issues	10	2.78
4	Chronic/Long-term illness	6	1.67
5	Severe non life-threatening illness	0	0
6	Life-threatening illness	0	0
7	Other	19	5.28
Sub-total		357	99.18
Missing		3	0.83
Total		360	100.0

"Other" comprised accidents, dental care (including teeth cleaning, scaling or extraction), contraception, pregnancy, immunization, vaccinations, work-related medical checkup, and sick certificates. Minor health issues included colds, influenza, and gastro-intestinal infections. The majority of Falun Gong respondents (89%, n=320) did not consult a medical practitioner during the six months prior to completing the survey. Less than 10% of Falun Gong respondents (9.8%, n=37) reported medical consultations. The two most common responses were "Minor health issues" and "Other." No Falun Gong respondents reported visiting medical practitioners for severe, non life-threatening, or life-threatening illnesses.

7.2.2 Item 38: Medical conditions before Falun Gong practice

Item 38 in HW1 asked Falun Gong respondents to specify any pre-existing medical condition(s) as diagnosed by medical practitioners before commencing Falun Gong practice. Findings indicated that Falun Gong respondents who reported pre-existing medical condition(s) had more health problems than non–Falun Gong respondents. Written responses were classified into four broad categories of medical conditions: 1) Mental health; 2) Muscularskeletal; 3) Respiratory; and 4) Other medical conditions. In Level 3, these broad medical categories were sorted into subcategories, as shown in Table 7.3.

Table 7.3 Three-level categorizing of medical conditions of Falun Gong respondents

Level 1: Meaning units	Level 2: Categories	Level 3: Subcategories
Respondents' written responses which included: asthma, depression, irregular period, stress, excessive thoughts, and attention deficit disorder	Mental health	• Anxiety disorder • Depression • Chronic fatigue • Mental health problems, such as psychoses, insomnia • Allergies/Hay fever • Asthma • Other respiratory conditions • Back (and neck) pain • Muscularskeletal • Chronic/Life-threatening • Gynecological conditions • Others

The creation of a subcategory was based on the frequency of that medical condition to enhance understanding of the findings. For instance, the mental health category was sub-categorized into anxiety disorder, depression, chronic fatigue, and miscellaneous mental health conditions. There were 21 reports for anxiety disorder, 17 for depression, 24 for chronic fatigue, and 21 miscellaneous mental health conditions.

Miscellaneous mental health conditions included nervous breakdown, psychoses or psychotic episodes, insomnia, and stress. Miscellaneous respiratory conditions encompassed bronchitis, cold, influenza, and sinusitis, while miscellaneous muscularskeletal conditions included arthritis, carpal tunnel syndrome, Guillain-Barré syndrome, multiple sclerosis, osteoarthritis, repetitive strain injury, rheumatoid arthritis, and scoliosis. Back (and neck) pain was categorised separately because of its frequency. Other medical conditions comprised chronic/life-threatening illnesses, gynaecological problems, and miscellaneous conditions.

In analyzing the data for this item, it was decided not to quantify the qualitative content in order to retain the richness and variety of Falun Gong respondents' self-reports to provide better insight into the health-wellness status of Falun Gong respondents before commencing Falun Gong practice. Due to the variety and numerous reports of multiple health problems, it was decided to categorize and report the frequency of all the different medical conditions instead of reporting the most severe or dominant medical condition of the 163 Falun Gong respondents' written responses. Reporting only the most severe medical condition would require a greater degree of researcher manipulation of the raw data, introduce subjectivity and involve making decisions for respondents as to what was most important and consequential for them.

Thus the decision to report all original medical conditions was made with the following intentions: 1) to be true to the self-reports of the respondents and to capture the true essence of their experience in the reporting and presentation of the data; 2) to manage subjectivity, minimize or eliminate researcher bias; and 3) to establish consistency, dependability and credibility, which are the fundamental characteristics of sound academic research (O'Leary, 2004).

Respondent 297 reported multiple medical health problems that could be classified into all of the four Level 2 categories of mental health, respiratory, musculoskeletal, and other medical conditions:

> *Incurable chronic conditions due to thyroid, adrenals, and pituitary gland (cause could not be identified). Also, severe allergies, degenerated discs causing loss of mobility and pain, sleep disorder, chronic fatigue, anxiety, etc. (Respondent 297).*

Likewise, Respondent 216 reported multiple health conditions: "Stomach ulcer, chronic headaches, fatigue, arthritis, incontinence, weakness on knees [sic], anxiety, and fear." Respondent 283 also indicated having multiple health problems and surgical procedures: "Arthritis, bronchitis, headache, urethritis, mastectomy, gastrostomy, and cholecystectomy." Approximately 50% of the 163 Falun Gong respondents (n=82) reported having two or more medical conditions. Table 7.4 shows the frequency of the medical conditions that Falun Gong respondents reported having prior to Falun Gong practice.

Table 7.4 Medical conditions before commencing Falun Gong practice

Level 2 Category		Level 3 Subcategory		Frequency
1	Mental health	•	Anxiety disorder	21
		•	Depression	17
		•	Chronic fatigue	24
		•	Miscellaneous	21
2	Musculoskeletal	•	Back (& neck) Pain	21
		•	Miscellaneous	29
3	Respiratory	•	Allergies/Hay fever	25
		•	Asthma	18
		•	Miscellaneous	26
4	Other	•	Chronic/Life-threatening illness	28
		•	Gynecological	12
		•	Miscellaneous	69

Chronic/life-threatening illnesses included five reports of cancer, 13 reports of heart disease, three reports of diabetes, five cases of hypertension, and two of hypotension. The cancers were breast cancer, cervical cancer, nose cancer, and skin cancer. A female respondent in her 70s (R283) reported multiple surgical procedures, including mastectomy, gastrostomy, and cholecystectomy. As there were more female (57.2%, n=207) than male respondents, a subcategory for gynecological conditions was added, involving cysts, irregular period, thrush, yeast infections, endometriosis, dysmenorrhea, menopausal symptoms, such as hot flushes, and one report of a major fibroid operation. Fifteen instances of gynecological conditions were listed, including the three reports of breast cancer, cervical cancer, and mastectomy classified in the Chronic/life-threatening category.

There were 69 reports of "Other Miscellaneous" (See Table 7.4), which comprised a variety of medical conditions, such as headaches, migraines, gastro-intestinal conditions (stomach ulcer and irritable bowel syndrome), eye and ear conditions, other chronic ailments, including kidney disease, hepatitis, hyperthyroidism, and hypothyroidism. One Falun Gong respondent (R289) reported multiple physical, mental health problems, and multiple medical conditions after a serious accident:

> ... coma (11 days), leaking of spinal fluid, fractured skull, damaged sinuses and broken jaw, broken wrists, cracked kneecap, deafness in the left ear, distorted vision, noise in my head, back and neck pain, osteoarthritis, loss of feeling in most of the left hand. Prior to the accident I had serious digestion problems, allergies, migraines, aches and pains, anxiety, and depression (Respondent 289).

Another respondent (R219) reported multiple medical conditions: "seasonal attacks of cold-cough-sinus congestion, retina-migraine, grand mal seizures [sic], indigestion, constipation, and diabetes in the family tree." A total of 45% of Falun Gong respondents (n=163) reported having specific pre-existing medical and health condition(s). Data from this item showed Falun Gong respondents were not very healthy individuals prior to commencing Falun Gong practice. Fifty percent of the 163 Falun Gong respondents (n=82) reported two or more pre-existing medical conditions, indicating they had poor health-wellness status before commencing Falun Gong practice.

7.2.3 Item 42: Initial attraction to Falun Gong

The Falun Gong respondents were provided with eight options to indicate what first attracted them to Falun Gong practice and asked to select three that most applied to them, without having to prioritize their selections. "Teachings of Falun Gong" was the most frequent choice, closely followed by "predestined relationship" and the "search for meaning in life." Table 7.5 shows the frequency and percentage distribution of respondents' selections in descending order.

Table 7.5 Initial attraction to Falun Gong

Option	Description	Frequency	Percent
4	Teachings of Falun Gong	182	50.6
7	A predestined relationship or *yuanfen* (e.g. "I knew this was for me.")	176	48.9
1	Search for meaning in life	172	47.8
5	Spiritual enlightenment offered by Falun Gong	136	37.8
6	Physical and mental health benefits	111	30.8
3	Falun Gong exercises	77	21.4
2	Family/friends practice Falun Gong	71	19.7
8	Other	28	7.8

7.2.4 Item 43: Other attractions of Falun Gong

To retain the essence, two levels of categorization and content analysis instead of three were used for the 27 written responses. Both levels of analysis were reported concurrently. Seventy percent of responses (n=19) comprised a phrase or one-sentence response. The responses were broadly categorized into comments that were similar to the themes in the listed options for Item 42 (see Table 7.5) and those that were different, which included curiosity, major turning points in life, positive regard for Falun Gong practitioners, teachings were free, Chinese Communist Party (CCP) persecution of Falun Gong, unusual encounters with Falun Gong, and miscellaneous comments, such as repaying karmic debt, affinity with traditional Chinese culture, and Falun Gong for youth and beauty. The following comments highlight some of these different themes:

7.2.4.1 Curiosity

I was very curious about why Falun Gong was so popular in China but banned by the CCP and would like to find the true story behind (Respondent 42).

*I was curious and after I was told it was a type of cultivation practice I liked
it even better (Respondent 110).*

*Curiosity. Initially, I was more interested to find out what Falun Gong is about
and all those news that were broadcasted from CCTV [sic] (Respondent 310).*

7.2.4.2 CCP persecution of Falun Gong

Initially I wanted to learn what the persecution was about. I knew if the regime
there was trying to cover it up, it must be something powerful (Respondent 195).

I felt that Falun Dafa must be a very powerful spiritual path to be so severely
persecuted by elements within the Chinese government! (Respondent 185).

7.2.4.3 Major turning points in life

Two Falun Gong respondents wrote about turning points in their life. A
young female respondent (R134) wrote, "I knew my life had to be changed
for [the] better and I felt that Falun Gong is the one to help me through." A
respondent in her fifties reminisced about her life journey:

> *My life changed dramatically midlife and I ventured in the many aspects
> of alternative/complementary therapies etc., which then led me into the
> metaphysical arena. Some years on I came upon Falun Gong, after having
> practiced tai chi, different forms of meditations, etc. Each step of this naturally
> unfolding journey in way and time led to the Fa [Falun Gong] and has
> revealed unexplainable and incredible realizations of my understandings
> of the cosmos, all of life and myself (Respondent 142).*

7.2.4.4 Positive regard of Falun Gong practitioners

Two Falun Gong respondents mentioned that the demeanor of Falun Gong
practitioners was what first attracted them to the practice:

> *The fact that all the practitioners I met were very nice and good people
> (Respondent 153).*

I wanted to know what exactly is Falun Gong because my friend is [a]
Falun Gong practitioner and he is so different from everyday person [sic]
(Respondent 251).

7.2.4.5 Teachings were free and encounters with Falun Gong

Respondent 303 was attracted to Falun Gong because the teachings were free of charge. Another respondent (R16) commented how their partner was "attracted by the energy and the fact that they weren't selling anything" and how the CCP anti–Falun Gong propaganda had the opposite impact on them.

A short time later we saw a [news] piece on CNN about the Zhongnanhai
incident with a Chinese government spokesperson criticizing the behavior of
the Falun Gong 'protestors' when the footage clearly showed their behavior
as exemplary. We were most impressed with such a silent and orderly
'protest.' We thought that if the Chinese Communist Party (CCP) was so
against Falun Gong then it was probably very good. We knew a lot about
the previous crimes of the CCP (Respondent 16).

7.2.4.6 Miscellaneous comments

Other respondents were initially attracted to Falun Gong for different reasons. One Falun Gong respondent (R185) mentioned "having a lifelong affinity with traditional Chinese culture and having learned Mandarin for three years," while another Falun Gong respondent stated that "it [Falun Gong] came from China – I was in an attraction to knowing everything about China phase."

Respondent 251 wondered, "if Falun Gong can help me solve the contradiction with my mother"? Another Falun Gong respondent (R234) indicated, "I was looking for a way to pay back debt incurred through doing the wrong thing" [sic]. And a female respondent (R356) wrote, "you can keep your youth and beauty by practicing Falun Gong."

The next two subsections report comments about reasons for the initial attraction to Falun Gong. Teachings of Falun Gong and health benefits were provided as options listed in Item 42 (See Table 7.5).

7.2.4.7 Teachings of Falun Gong

Several Falun Gong respondents referred to the profundity of the teachings as their first attraction to Falun Gong. One respondent (R347) described "Master's teachings [as] very powerful and relevant," while Respondent 303 alluded to "the balance of mind and body" and Falun Gong's universal principles of truthfulness, compassion and forbearance. Respondent 142 reported that the teachings of Falun Gong "revealed unexplainable and incredible realizations of my understandings of the cosmos, all of life and myself." Another respondent (R321) reported how "over time, with continual reading of *Zhuan Falun,* I found an inner wisdom and profound truth that I could not turn my back on."

7.2.4.8 Health benefits and perceived self-improvement

Respondent 195 reported looking for a practice "to build internal energy and none of the martial arts had what I was looking for," while another (R211) stated that family members' illnesses had first attracted them to Falun Gong. Three respondents reported the following:

> I was looking for some form of exercise to improve my health and joined Falun Gong exercise "by chance" i.e. just join in the practice without any knowledge of what it was all about [sic] (Respondent 32).

> I was looking for some type of qigong to learn and saw people practicing Falun Gong near my house and so I joined in (Respondent 48).

> It was suggested to me that it could help my condition. I had problems moving around, double vision, etc. I tried it on the off chance that it would help, having tried many other things. Upon watching the Falun Gong video, I suddenly felt better than I had in a long time. I decided that I would give it a shot, and in a month (arguably up to three months) I was 100% [sic] (Respondent 182).

This concludes the qualitative content reporting for Item 43 that asked respondents to specify what first attracted them to Falun Gong. The Falun Gong respondents who provided comments came from diverse ethnic backgrounds, from Chinese-Malaysians and Indian to mostly Caucasians born in different countries.

7.2.5 Item 44: How Falun Gong led to better health and wellness

The Falun Gong respondents were given eight options and asked to select three that most applied to them on how Falun Gong practice led to better health and wellness in their life. Respondents were not required to prioritize their selections. Table 7.6 displays the frequency and percentage distribution of their selections in descending order.

Table 7.6 How Falun Gong led to better health and wellness

Option	Description	Frequency	Percent
6	Improving *xinxing* or moral character based on the principles of truthfulness, compassion and forbearance	328	91.1
2	Regular study of Falun Gong teachings	280	77.8
1	Falun Gong exercise routine	170	47.2
5	Positive change of attitude towards life since practicing Falun Gong	158	43.9
4	Improved stress coping ability	51	14.2
7	Falun Gong experience sharing conferences	24	6.7
3	Falun Gong community	18	5.0
8	Other	5	1.4

The majority of Falun Gong respondents selected "improving *xinxing* or moral character based on the principles of truthfulness, compassion, and forbearance."

7.2.6 Other reasons for Falun Gong leading to better health and wellness

The Falun Gong respondents were asked in Item 45 of the HW1 to specify other reasons for how Falun Gong had led to better health and wellness in their life. As there were only seven written comments, it was unnecessary to use the three-level procedure. The researcher reported the qualitative content verbatim to retain the essence of the seven respondents' written comments in Table 7.7.

Table 7.7 Other reasons for Falun Gong leading to better health and wellness

Assigned ID	Falun Gong respondents' written comments
R12	Gave life a meaning
R98	Help in the improving in the overall wellness of society [sic]
R142	I can relate to each one of the above aspects of Falun Gong in having a pivotal role in my overall health and wellbeing
R150	Regular study of Falun Gong teachings
R182	Incredible change in perspective, namely seeing the bigger picture of situations as opposed to focusing on own needs. This was not a one-time occurrence but an enlargement of perspective that has been happening regularly since I started to practice
R196	Body purification by *Shifu*
R213	Experience sharing

Comments from Respondents 150 and 213 were identical to the listed options provided for Item 44, displayed in Table 7.6. "Experience sharing" refers to both formal experience-sharing conferences and informal group or person-to-person sharing among Falun Gong practitioners.

Respondent 182 mentioned insights gleaned from Falun Gong teachings, not being self-focused and considering others first as leading to better health and wellness. "Body purification" refers to the body purification process associated with Falun Gong practice as discussed in the book *Zhuan Falun* (H. Li, 2001b, pp. 3, 6, 40). *Shifu*, a Chinese term for master, refers to Mr. Li Hongzhi, the founder of Falun Gong. This completes the qualitative content reporting for Falun Gong respondents.

7.3 Written comments from non–Falun Gong respondents

This section reports the qualitative data for Item 13 in Section 2 of HW2 relating to reasons for medical visits for non–Falun Gong respondents.

Non–Falun Gong respondents consulted medical practitioners more often than Falun Gong respondents.

7.3.1 Item 13: Reason for medical visits by non–Falun Gong respondents

Written responses of non–Falun Gong respondents were analyzed and processed following the same procedure as described for Falun Gong respondents in Section 7.2.1. The qualitative content was sorted into seven categories. Where there were two or more medical conditions from the same respondent, they were categorized by the most severe medical condition. For example, a multiple case with knee problems, arthritis, atrial fibrillation, and heart failure was classified as Category 6 (life-threatening illness). "Other" in Category 7 comprised reasons such as accidents, dental care (including teeth cleaning, scaling or tooth extraction), contraception, pregnancy, immunization, vaccinations, work-related medical checkups, and sick certificates. Minor health issues included colds, influenza and gastro-intestinal infections. Table 7.8 shows the frequency and percentage distribution for reason for medical visits by non–Falun Gong respondents.

Table 7.8 Reasons for medical visits by non–Falun Gong respondents

Category	Description	Frequency	Percent
1	None/Not applicable	71	30.9
2	Routine medical checkup	26	11.3
3	Minor health issues	73	31.7
4	Chronic/Long-term illness	27	11.7
5	Severe non life-threatening illness	9	3.9
6	Life-threatening illness	3	1.3
7	Other	18	7.8
Sub-total		227	98.7
Missing		3	1.3
Total		230	100.0

A total of 68% of non–Falun Gong respondents (n=156) consulted medical practitioners compared to 10% of Falun Gong respondents (n=37). Thirty-one percent of non–Falun Gong respondents (n=71) did not visit any medical practitioners compared to 89% of Falun Gong respondents (n=320). More non–Falun Gong respondents (32%, n=73) reported consulting a medical practitioner for minor health problems than Falun Gong respondents (2.8%, n=10). There were nine reports of severe, non life-threatening illness and three life-threatening cases from non–Falun Gong respondents, whereas there were none from Falun Gong respondents. The three life-threatening cases were atrial fibrillation and heart failure, concussion, and ovarian cancer. Non–Falun Gong respondents reported 47 instances of two or more listings compared to three cases from Falun Gong respondents.

Overall, non–Falun Gong respondents had more medical conditions than Falun Gong respondents and visited their medical practitioners more often than Falun Gong respondents. This completes the reporting of all qualitative content analysis for Falun Gong and non–Falun Gong respondents.

CHAPTER 8

Comparison Between Groups

8.1 Chapter overview

This chapter presents tabulated summary of comparisons between Falun Gong and non–Falun Gong respondents. Findings from this research indicated that the two groups share many similarities in their demographic profiles. Despite similar demographic characteristics, there were observed differences in the medical history, health-wellness self-reports, and general health statuses between Falun Gong and non–Falun Gong respondents. These similarities and differences are summarized and presented in descriptive tables in this chapter.

8.2 Demographic similarities between the two groups

Overall, Falun Gong respondents were mainly females, married, from diverse ethnic backgrounds, had tertiary education qualifications, and a professional career. They were mainly Chinese/Asians whose first language is not English. Most of them resided in Australia and New Zealand, or Canada and United States. Non–Falun Gong respondents were also mainly females, married, from diverse ethnic backgrounds, with tertiary education qualifications and a professional career. However, they were more likely to have English as their first language and resided in Australia and New Zealand or Canada and United States.

The similarities in the demographic profiles between Falun Gong and non–Falun Gong respondents are summarized in Table 8.1. Italics are used for the non–Falun Gong data to highlight observed differences between the two groups.

8.3 Health-wellness differences between the two groups

While Falun Gong and non–Falun Gong respondents shared similar demographics, there was a contrast between the two groups in their medical history, self-perceptions of their health and general health-wellness statuses. Overall, Falun Gong respondents reported very healthy lifestyle habits and experienced better health-wellness than non–Falun Gong respondents. Most did not visit medical practitioners, took no medications, and spent very little money on medical and health expenses. Nearly all were non-smokers, did not drink alcohol or use recreational drugs.

Non–Falun Gong respondents were healthy with moderate lifestyle habits. They consulted medical practitioners more often, took more medication, remedies and supplements, and spent more money on medical expenses and health supplements than Falun Gong respondents. Nearly 50% of those who consumed alcohol or used recreational drugs reported no plans to stop. Table 8.2 displays a summary of the medical history, visits to medical practitioner, medication intake, medical, and health expenses between Falun Gong and non–Falun Gong respondents.

Chart 8.2 and Chart 8.3 present a visual comparison of the differences between the two groups for cigarette smoking, alcohol consumption and recreational drug use.

Table 8.1 Summary of demographic profile of the two groups

	Falun Gong respondents	Non–Falun Gong respondents
Gender	More females (57%, n=206) than males (42%, n=151, missing=3)	More females (63%, n=146) than males (35%, n=81, missing=3)
Age Range	Mode: 30-39 years (26%, n=93, missing=2); Mean: 3.72	Mode: 20-29 years & 50-59 years age range (22%, n=51, missing=2); Mean: 3.74
Marital status	Mostly married: (61%, n=218); Never married: (24%, n=85), the 2nd highest group; De facto: (1.4%, n=5, missing=2)	Mostly married: (48%, n=110); Never married: (31%, n=72) the 2nd highest group; De facto: (8.3, n=19, missing=2)
Ethnicity	Diverse: 37 ethnicities identified	Diverse: 33 ethnicities identified
Country of Birth	45 countries identified: Highest: mainland China (28%, n=97); 2nd: Asia (24%, n=86); 3rd: Australia & NZ (19%, n=68);4th: Canada/US (13%, n=46)	37 countries identified: Highest: Australia & NZ (n=92, 40%) 2nd: Asia (21%, n=48); 3rd: mainland China (10%, n=23); 4th: Canada/US (10%, n=22)
Country of Residence	Most resided in Australia & NZ (43%, n=154); 2nd: Canada/US (32%, n=114); 3rd: Asia (14%, n=51)	Most resided in Australia and New Zealand (66%, n=151) 2nd: Canada /US (15%, n=35); 3rd: Asia (12%, n=26)
English: First Language	"No" English is not: (63%, n=226); "Yes" English is: (35%, n=128) Mandarin or Chinese dialects, for example Cantonese, Hakka, & Shanghainese: (44%, n=164)	"No" English is not: 41% (n=94); "Yes" English is: 57% (n=130); Mandarin or Chinese dialects, for example Cantonese & Hokkien: (23%, n=53)
Highest Education	Mode: undergraduate degree: (33%, n=117, missing=5) Second: High School (29%, n=105) Master's degree or PhD/Doctorate: (30%, n=107)	Mode: undergraduate degree (34%, n=79, missing=6) Second: High School (32%, n=74) Master's degree or PhD/Doctorate: (16%, n=36)
Occupation (Top 3)	1st: Business/computer information technology (15%, n=54) 2nd: Arts, media, social sciences, and misc. professionals (15%, n=54) 3rd: Clerical, sales, administrative & service workers (12%, n=43)	1st: Business/computer information technology (n=36, 16%) 2nd: Clerical, sales, admin and service workers (14%, n=33) 3rd: Retired/Home Duties (14%, n=31)

Table 8.2 Summary of medical history and health status of the two groups

	Falun Gong respondents	Non–Falun Gong respondents
Doctor Visit	88% (n=316, missing=6) did not consult a physician. 8.3% (n=30) consulted a physician 3 times during the 6 months prior to completing survey.	28% (n=65, missing=4) did not consult a physician. 55% (n=127) consulted a physician 1-3 times during the 6 months prior to completing this survey.
Reason for Visit	Falun Gong respondents had fewer medical conditions: Medical checkup (0.6%, n=2); Minor health issues (2.8%, n=10); Chronic/long-term illness (1.7%, n=6); Severe non life-threatening or life-threatening illness: None.	Non–Falun Gong respondents had more medical conditions: Medical checkup (11%, n=26); Minor health issues (32%, n=73); Chronic/long-term illness (12%, n=27); Severe non life-threatening (4%, n=9); Life-threatening (1.3%, n=3)
Use of Medication and Supplements	95% (n=341, missing=4) did not use any form of medication, homeopathic remedies, multi-vitamins or health supplements. Prescription: (1.9%, n=7); Over counter drugs: (0.3%, n=1); Chinese herbs: 0%; Western herbs: (0.3%, n=1); Homeopathic: (0.3%, n=1); Vitamins & supplements: (1.4%, n=5)	35% (n=81, missing=8) did not use any form of medication, homeopathic remedies, multi-vitamins or health supplements. Most used a mix of medication & remedies. Prescription: (32%, n=74); Over counter drugs: (16.5%, n=38); Chinese herbs: (5.6%, n=13); Western herbs: (3%, n=7); Homeopathic: (4%, n=9); Vitamins & supplements: (29%, n=66)
Medical Health Expenses	8% (n=30) spent money on medical and health expenses. 92% (n=330) did not spend any money in this way.	67% (n=153) spent money on medical and health expenses. 33% of non–Falun Gong respondents (n=77) did not spend money in this way.
Cigarette Smoking	98% (n=352, missing=3) do not smoke cigarettes.	86% (n=198, missing=5) do not smoke cigarettes. .
Alcohol Consumption	97% (n=349, missing=3) did not consume alcohol. 2% (n=8) reported YES to consuming alcohol.	37% (n=85, missing=7) did not drink alcohol, 60% (n=138) reported YES. Of those who consume alcohol, over half had no plans to stop.
Recreational Drug Use	No recreational drug use: (99.7%, n=355, missing=4)	No recreational drug use: (92%, n=211, missing=11); 3.5% (n=8) reported YES. Of those who reported taking recreational drugs, 4 had no plans to stop.

Chart 8.1 Cigarette smoking – Falun Gong (T) compared to non–Falun Gong respondents (B)

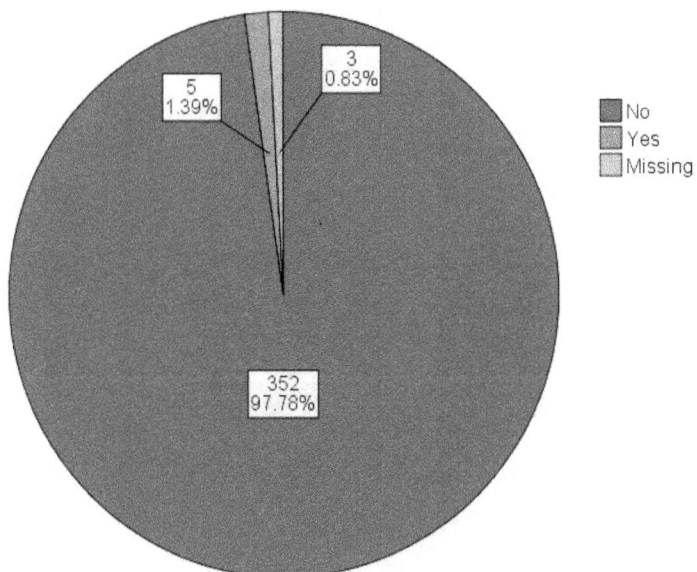

Cigarette Smoking: 1=No; 2=Yes

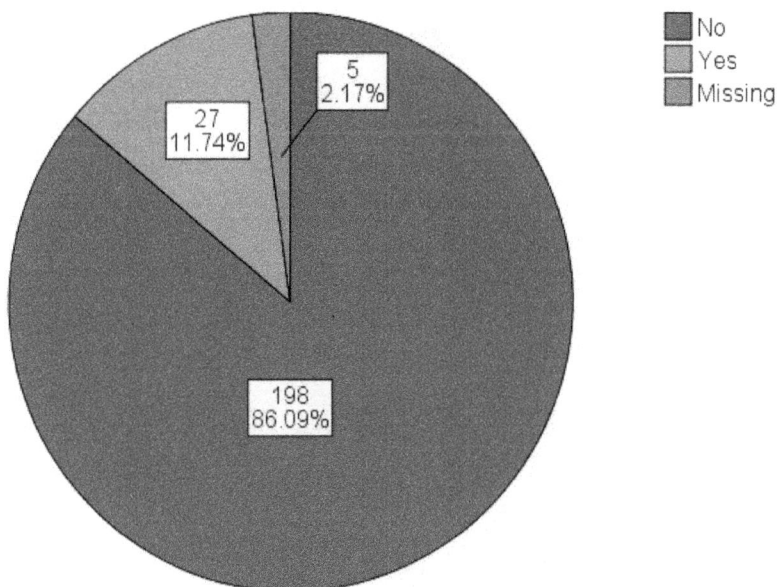

Cigarette Smoking: 1=No; 2=Yes

Chart 8.2 Alcohol consumption – Falun Gong (T) *compared to non–Falun Gong respondents* (B)

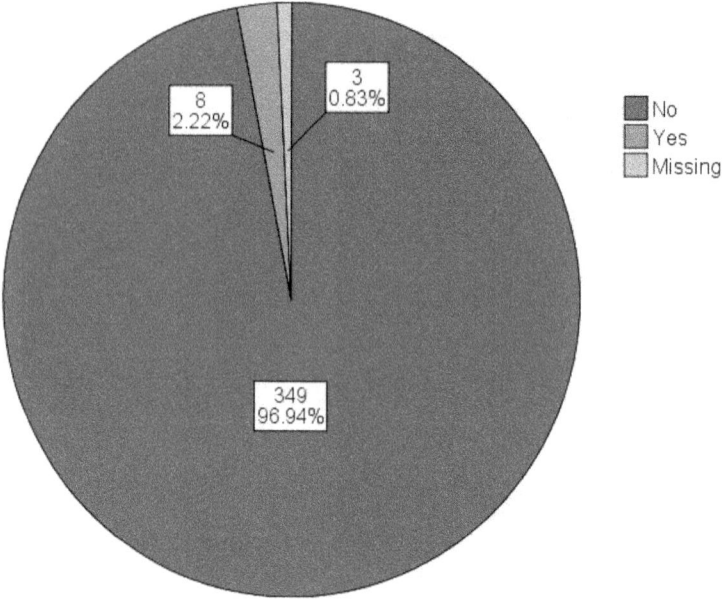

Alcohol Consumption: 1=No; 2=Yes

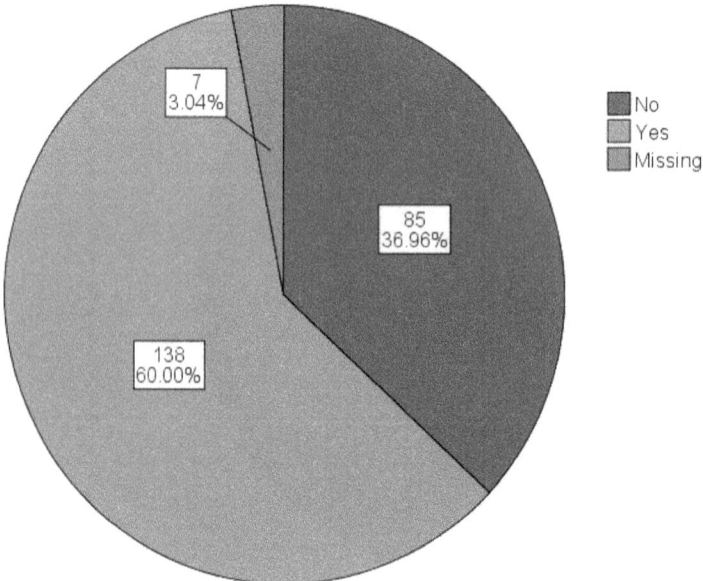

Alcohol Consumption: 1=No; 2=Yes

Chart 8.3 Recreational drug use – Falun Gong (T) *compared to non–Falun Gong respondents* (B)

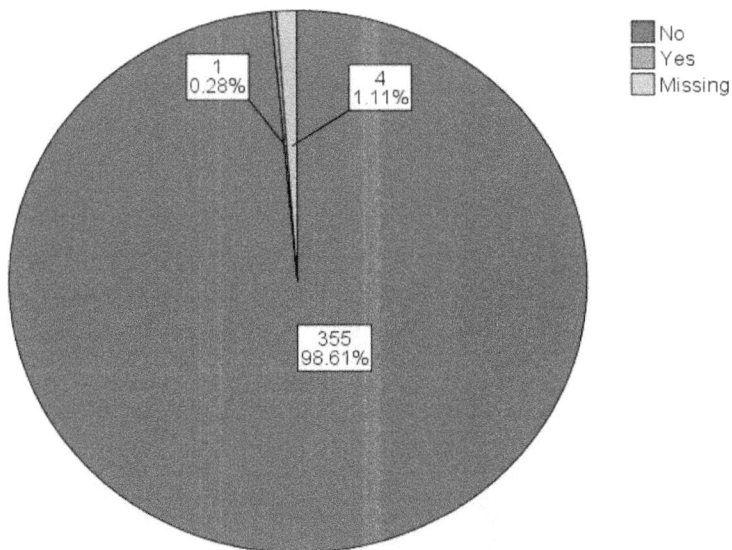

Recreational Drug Use: 1=No; 2=Yes

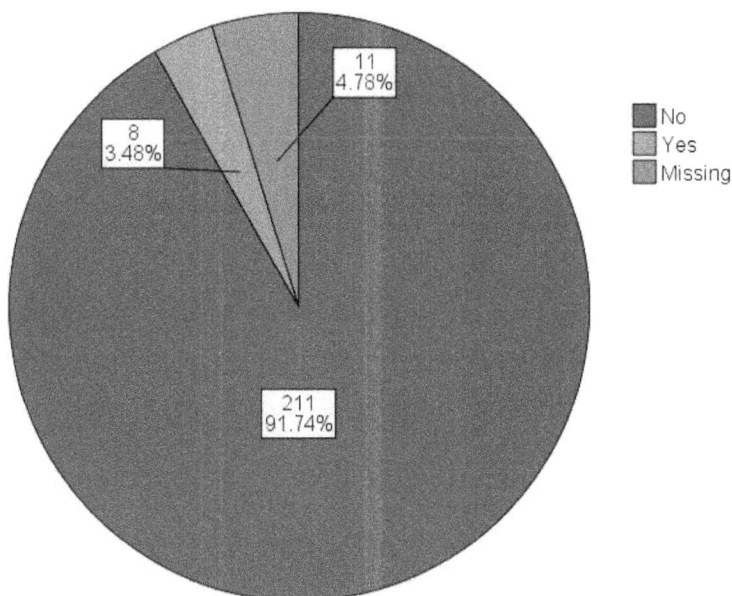

Recreational Drug Use: 1=No; 2=Yes

8.4 Comparison between groups for the SF-36

Findings for the SF-36 Health Survey for Falun Gong respondents and non–Falun Gong respondents groups were reported separately in Chapter 5 and Chapter 6 of this book. This section presents a descriptive summary of comparisons between the two groups for the SF-36 and also the Pearson chi-square calculations, which were done for the SF-36 items to verify whether the differences between the two groups were statistically significant or not. Findings were analyzed with SPSS (Version 15) software program with the valid data, which excluded missing data. For instance, chi-square test for general health status (Item 1) is $\chi^2(4, n= 581) = 149.51$, $p<0.001$. The results from the Pearson chi-square test for all the SF-36 items are presented in Table 8.3.

Table 8.3 Pearson chi-square tests for all items in the SF-36 Health Survey

Items description	χ^2 value	df	p value
General health status	149.51	4	0.001
General health one year ago	69.19	4	0.001
Physical health limits daily activities			
Vigorous activities	58.34	2	0.001
Moderate activities	55.40	2	0.001
Lift/carry groceries	37.76	2	0.001
Climb several stairs	70.48	2	0.001
Climb one flight of stairs	37.28	3	0.001
Bend, kneel or stoop	58.49	2	0.001
Walk more than a mile	47.43	2	0.001
Walk several blocks	34.59	2	0.001
Walk one block	25.23	2	0.001
Bathe or dress yourself	16.72	2	0.001
Problems with work due physical health			
Reduce work time	18.70	1	0.001
Do less than you like	41.31	1	0.001
Limited in work or activities	29.74	1	0.001
Difficulty doing work	27.01	1	0.001
Problems with work due emotional health			
Reduce work time	34.29	1	0.001

Items description	χ^2 value	df	p value
Do less than you like	24.84	1	0.001
Did not do work as carefully as usual	21.93	1	0.001
Extent physical/emotional issues affect social life	58.83	3	0.001
Physical pain during the past four weeks	32.56	4	0.001
Pain affecting work	54.75	4	0.001
Positive feelings and how things had been			
Full of life	74.83	5	0.001
Calm and peaceful	131.43	5	0.001
A lot of energy	121.56	5	0.001
Happy person	44.657	5	0.001
Negative feelings and how things had been			
Very nervous	34.94	5	0.001
Down in the dumps	42.77	5	0.001
Downhearted and blue	56.17	5	0.001
Worn out	148.36	5	0.001
Tired	106.98	5	0.001
Time physical/emotional pbms affect social activities	67.10	4	0.001
Perceptions of their health-wellness status			
I seem to get sick a little easier than other people	120.28	4	0.001
I expect my health to get worse	200.93	4	0.001
I am as healthy as anybody I know	69.59	4	0.001
My health is excellent	196.07	4	0.001

Pearson chi-square results indicated that the differences between Falun Gong and non–Falun Gong respondents were all statistically significant at p=<0.001. There is a one-in-a-thousand probability that the difference in their health-wellness status is due to chance alone, which suggests that Falun Gong could be the reason for the health-wellness differences between Falun Gong and non–Falun Gong respondents.

However, findings cannot ascertain a causal link between Falun Gong practice and health-wellness effect. It is beyond the aim and scope of this research to examine other variables or factors that could cause a health-wellness difference between the two groups. Nonetheless, it can be suggested that Falun Gong has a positive health-wellness effect and that the practice elicits a more positive self-perceived health-wellness status for Falun Gong respondents. Table 8.4 highlights the observed differences between the two groups for some of the items in the SF-36, such as respondents' general health status and perceptions of their health-wellness status.

Table 8.4 Highlights of differences between Falun Gong and non–Falun Gong respondents for the SF-36 Health Survey

Item	Falun Gong respondents	Non–Falun Gong respondents
General Health Status	Excellent=53% (n=192)	Excellent=10% (n=24)
Physical Health Limits Daily Activities	Vigorous activities: Not limited at all=73% (n=261)	Vigorous activities: Not limited at all=41% (n=94)
	Moderate activities: Not limited at all=93% (n=333)	Moderate activities: Not limited at all=68% (n=157)
	Climb several stairs: Not limited at all=87% (n=314)	Climb several stairs: Not limited at all=58% (n=133)
	Bend, kneel or stoop: Not limited at all=91% (n=328)	Bend, kneel or stoop: Not limited at all=65% (n=150)
	Work more than a mile: Not limited at all=91% (n=326)	Work more than a mile: Not limited at all=68% (n=157)
Extent Phy / Emotional Issues Affect Social Life	Not at all=83% (n=297) Slightly=14% (n=51); Moderately=1.4% (n=5)	Not at all=56% (n=128); Slightly=27% (n=62); Moderately=11% (n=25)
Positive Feelings and how things had been	Full of Life: 81% (n=293) all or most of the time	Full of Life: 55% (n=127) all or most of the time
	Calm and Peaceful: 83% (n=298) all or most of the time	Calm and Peaceful: 44% (n=102) all or most of the time
	A Lot of Energy: 82% (n=294) all or most of the time	A Lot of Energy: 44% (n=100) all or most of the time
	Happy Person: 84% (n=303) all or most of the time	Happy Person: 64% (n=147) all or most of the time

Item	Falun Gong respondents	Non–Falun Gong respondents
Negative Feelings and how things had been	Very Nervous: 86% (n=308) None / little of the time Down in the dumps: 73% (n=262) None of the time Downhearted/Blue: 92% (n= 330) None / little of the time Worn out: 87% (n=312) None / little of the time Tired: 78% (n=279) None / little of the time	Very Nervous: 71% (n=162) None / little of the time Down in the dumps: 49% (n=113) None of the time Downhearted/Blue: 69% (n=159) None / little of the time Worn out: 43% (n=98) None / little of the time Tired: 39% (n=89) None / little of the time
Time Phy & Emotional Problems Affect Social Life	None of the time: (81%, n=292) More respondents reported that physical and emotional problems did not affect their social activities.	None of the time: (51%, n=118) Fewer respondents reported that physical and emotional issues affected their social activities.
Perceptions of their Health-wellness Status	Definitely false statements: "I seem to get sick a little easier than other people." (87%, n=313) "I expect my health to get worse." (90%, n=324) Definitely true statements: "I am as healthy as anybody I know." (65%, n=234) "My health is excellent." (76%, n=274)	Definitely false statements: "I seem to get sick a little easier than other people." (47%, n=108) "I expect my health to get worse." (36.5%, n=84) Definitely true statements: "I am as healthy as anybody I know." (31%, n=72) "My health is excellent." (19%, n=44)
Summary	Overall, Falun Gong respondents' self-perceived general health reports were excellent and much more positive than non–Falun Gong respondents.	Overall, non–Falun Gong respondents' self-perceived general health reports were not as good or as positive as Falun Gong respondents.

8.5 Summary

Chapter 8 completes the comparison of findings between the Falun Gong respondents and non–Falun Gong respondents. Findings from Part A of the research revealed many demographic similarities between Falun Gong and non–Falun Gong respondents. However, there are observed differences between Falun Gong and non–Falun Gong respondents in their medical history, self-perceptions of their health, and their general health-wellness statuses. Findings indicated that while non–Falun Gong respondents were healthy individuals, those who practice Falun Gong experienced better health-wellness outcomes than those who did not practice Falun Gong. Falun Gong respondents were more likely to report excellent health, display more optimistic self-perception and a more positive regard for their health-wellness status. Pearson chi-square analysis indicated that the differences were statistically significant between the two groups for the SF-36 items.

CHAPTER 9

Analysis and Discussion

It's known that what actually causes people to become ill is seventy percent psychological and thirty percent physiological. (H. Li, 2001b, p. 218).

9.1 Chapter overview

This chapter presents the analysis and discussion of the findings of this research. It endeavors to provide insight into possible differences between Falun Gong and non–Falun Gong respondents and the health-wellness effects of Falun Gong. The findings are discussed with reference to Falun Gong and how it may contribute to better health and wellness in individuals who practice it, and provide insights into its potential for health and wellness. As mentioned in previous chapters, the aims of this research were to obtain a demographic profile of Falun Gong respondents, investigate the health-wellness effects of Falun Gong as perceived by Falun Gong practitioners, and to determine whether individuals who practice Falun Gong experience better health-wellness than those who do not.

Findings indicated that there are observed similarities between Falun Gong and non–Falun Gong respondents and statistically significant differences in health-wellness status between Falun Gong and non–Falun Gong respondents as indicated in previous chapters. This analysis and discussion will hopefully contribute to a better understanding of Falun Gong and its health-wellness effects on those who practice it. However, readers must keep in mind that the discussion is based on the findings of this survey. Greater knowledge of and insight into the teachings and practice of Falun Gong can only be obtained through reading the teachings of Falun Gong and conducting more in-depth studies into the lived experiences of Falun Gong practitioners.

9.2 Overview of findings

Findings from Part A of the research revealed similar demographic characteristics between Falun Gong and non–Falun Gong respondents. In contrast, findings from Part B of the research indicated that while non–Falun Gong respondents were healthy individuals, those who practice Falun Gong experienced even better health and wellness than those who did not. Falun Gong respondents consulted medical practitioners less frequently, took no or less medication or health supplements, and spent much less on medical and health expenses compared to non–Falun Gong respondents. Falun Gong respondents also reported fewer medical conditions or reasons for consulting medical practitioners, in sharp contrast to their self-reports of numerous medical conditions prior to commencing Falun Gong practice. The statistically significant differences between Falun Gong and non–Falun Gong respondents were revealed in their general health self-reports with Falun Gong respondents reporting better, more positive and excellent general health-wellness status.

9.2.1 Similarities in demographic profile

Given that non–Falun Gong respondents comprised family members and friends invited by Falun Gong respondents to participate in the survey, similarities in demographic profile was anticipated, although it was possible that the two groups could have been different. Non–Falun Gong respondents were either a spouse, parent, sister, brother, aunt, uncle, cousin, friend, work colleague, or neighbor who lived or worked together, and typically shared similar backgrounds and life situations with Falun Gong respondents because of their proximity to each other. In having family and friends of Falun Gong respondents as the comparison group, the researcher aimed to establish some common characteristics between the two groups in order to ascertain whether, despite their similar home or work environment and proximity to each other, one group would emerge as the variant in terms of health-wellness effects. The researcher acknowledges that there are other factors to consider, such as the halo effect (Oh & Ramaprasad, 2003; Thorndike, 1920), the Hawthorne Effect (M. Chiesa & Hobbs, 2008; Hindle, 2008; McCarney et al., 2007; Oxford Dictionary, 2005; VandenBos, 2007), and the social desirability effect (Booth-Kewley et al., 2007; Heerwegh, 2009; Tourangeau et al., 2003; VandenBos, 2007) that could influence the findings of this research.

9.2.2 Gender distribution and why there were more female respondents

Gender distribution indicated that there were more female than male respondents. This finding is consistent with the combined results of mainland China health surveys that indicated a gender distribution of 72.9% female versus 27.1% male (Authors Unknown, 2002; D. Palmer, 2007). It is also consistent with studies conducted outside of mainland China by Ownby (2003b; 2008a), S. J. Palmer (2003) and Falun Gong practitioners in North America (Authors Unknown, 1999, 2003a) although there were no clear explanations for this occurrence. Findings indicated that there were more females than males for both Falun Gong and non–Falun Gong respondents. It is possible that female Falun Gong respondents have more female non–Falun Gong friends and family members willing to complete the HW2 than non–Falun Gong respondents. Another possibility could be that women are more spiritual, more receptive to alternative, Eastern mind-body meditative movement practices, such as yoga, tai chi and meditation, and perhaps more open to completing a health-wellness survey.

The literature review in Chapter 2 indicated that more women than men reported using complementary and alternative medicine (CAM) (Barnes et al., 2004; Upchurch et al., 2007), and more educated Asian American women preferred CAM therapies (Mehta et al., 2007). Upchurch et al. (2007) revealed that women were more receptive to the benefits of integrating CAM with conventional medical treatment and more willing to try something different. Women are "often the managers of health care within the family" (Upchurch et al., 2007, p. 103), a role that fits in with traditional social roles of the woman as the principal carer and nurturer of the family, while the man goes out to work and economically supports the family.

Data from over seven decades of Gallup surveys indicated that women were more inclined to higher religiosity/spirituality than men (Gallup Jr., 2002; Winseman, 2002a, 2002b, 2003). Some of the reasons given for this gender difference included traditional, social, and cultural roles of women as the mothers, carers, nurturers of the family, and multifaceted differences in the female and male consciousness (Gallup Jr., 2002). Women were more religious, more spiritually committed than men (Gallup Jr., 2002; Winseman, 2002a,

2002b, 2003), and more inclined to use mind-body therapies and practice yoga, and other meditative movement practices (Barnes et al., 2004; Mehta et al., 2007; Upchurch et al., 2007), which reflects the propensity for more female involvement in Falun Gong.

9.2.3 Age range

The average age range of both groups was located between the 30 to 39 years and 40 to 49 years age range, closer towards the 40 to 49 years age range. This is not a definitive average age but it is indicative that the average age of respondents is below 50, comparable with the average age of Falun Gong respondents in three different North American studies: 1) by Ownby (2003b; 2008a) and S. J. Palmer (2003) that had a mean of 42 years; 2) by Porter (2003) with a mean of 37 years; and 3) by North American Falun Gong practitioners with a mean of 38.9 years (Authors Unknown, 1999, 2003a). The average age of Falun Gong practitioners outside of mainland China is thus relatively younger (below 50 years old) than those in the mainland China surveys, which reported that over 62% of the total sample size from the five mainland China health surveys were above 50 years old (Authors Unknown, 1999). This younger age phenomenon could be the result of immigration laws in destination countries like Australia, New Zealand, Canada, and the United States, which favor and grant student or permanent resident visas to younger and more highly educated individuals. Falun Gong in North America was described as "a product of recent Chinese immigration" (Ownby, 2008a), which could be the same for Falun Gong in Australia and New Zealand.

9.2.4 Ethnicity

Both Falun Gong and non–Falun Gong respondents came from diverse racial and cultural backgrounds. A total of 37 and 33 ethnicities were identified for Falun Gong and non–Falun Gong groups respectively. The global ethnic profile of Falun Gong respondents is different to Falun Gong respondents in North America, which Ownby (2003b) described as "overwhelmingly Chinese" (p. 308) (91% ethnic Chinese) with a sprinkle of Westerners (9%) described as non-conforming "spiritual seekers," or "Western hippies" (p. 309). Fewer than half the Falun Gong respondents (47%, n=170) from this research were ethnic Chinese, while 24% (n=86) identified themselves as Caucasians. The exact total figure was difficult to establish as some respondents identified themselves as Anglo-Celtic, Greeks, Italians, Polish, Russians, etc., while others by their nationality such as Canadians, Americans, with eight percent of Falun Gong respondents (n=27) identifying themselves as Australians. Findings from this research indicated that the global demographic profile of Falun Gong is changing, with respondents coming from diverse ethnic and multicultural backgrounds.

This research found that the global demographic profile of Falun Gong respondents was not predominantly mainland Chinese. Only 28% of Falun Gong respondents (n=97) were born in mainland China, with 24% (n=86) born in Asia and not necessarily of ethnic Chinese origin. The demographic profile of Falun Gong respondents from this research can therefore be described as more multi-ethnic and multicultural than other studies, a characteristic that was observed in the South Australian Falun Gong community where Caucasians, Asians (Malaysian, Cambodian and Vietnamese) and other ethnic groups often outnumbered mainland Chinese practitioners in many group activities (Thompson, 2009). This could be due to the spread of Falun Gong outside of mainland China to involve individuals from other and different ethnic and cultural backgrounds. It could also be that Ownby-Palmer's (Ownby, 2003b, 2008a; S. J. Palmer, 2003) field studies were conducted in 2000-2001, just after the onset of the persecution of Falun Gong in mainland China by the Chinese Communist Party (CCP) in July 1999 and in the early stages of Falun Gong development outside of mainland China, whereas data collection for this research occurred in 2007 when Falun Gong outside of mainland China was more established and had spread to different parts of the world. Ownby-Palmer's field studies were restricted to specific cities/regions in Canada and the U.S., whereas this research involved an online survey available to a more diverse range of respondents from different parts of the world. The online survey was in English, requiring computer and Internet access, and likely to attract more English-speaking respondents with computer skills and Internet access.

9.2.5 Highest education level

Another similarity between the Falun Gong and non–Falun Gong group was their highest education level. The mode for both groups was an undergraduate degree held by 33% of Falun Gong respondents (n=117) and three percent of non–Falun Gong respondents (n=79). However, there were more Falun Gong respondents (30%, n=107) with master's, PhDs, or doctoral degrees than non–Falun Gong respondents (16%, n=36). Nonetheless, respondents from both groups were well educated with business/finance or computer information technology as their most popular occupation. This profile of Falun Gong respondents was consistent with the results from other Falun Gong studies outside of mainland China by Ownby (2003b; 2008a) and Falun Gong practitioners in North America (Authors Unknown, 1999, 2003a).

In summary, Falun Gong and non–Falun Gong respondents shared many observed similar demographic characteristics. They lived or worked together or typically shared similar backgrounds and life situations because of their proximity and relationship with each other. Demographic data was consistent in many instances with studies conducted in mainland China, as well as those outside of mainland China.

9.3 Differences between Falun Gong and non–Falun Gong respondents

Some of the differences in characteristics between the two groups are discussed in the following subsections.

9.3.1 Difference in the sample size

The total sample size (n=590) comprised 360 Falun Gong respondents and 230 non–Falun Gong respondents. This could indicate that 130 Falun Gong respondents did not invite a non–Falun Gong respondent, or they did not know anyone they could ask, or that the person they asked did not complete the HW2. It is possible that some Falun Gong respondents may not have had friends outside their own Falun Gong circle or community that they felt comfortable to invite to participate in the research. Like different ethnic groups or Christian communities, it is likely that Falun Gong respondents tend to socialize within their own community (Court, 2007). Falun Gong respondents were not required to invite a non–Falun Gong respondent to participate in the survey. See Appendix 2 for the RIS. The discrepancy in numbers between the two groups did not influence the findings.

9.3.2 Country of birth versus country of residence

More than half of the Falun Gong respondents (52%, n=183) were born in mainland China or in Asian countries such as Malaysia, Singapore, Indonesia, Philippines, Thailand, and Vietnam, whereas 40% of non–Falun Gong respondents (n=92) were born in Australia and New Zealand and only 10% of non–Falun Gong respondents (n=23) were born in mainland China. A total of 45 and 37 different countries of birth were identified for Falun Gong and non–Falun Gong groups respectively, indicating the diversity of their country of origin.

Although both Falun Gong and non–Falun Gong respondents were born in many different countries, the majority resided predominantly in two main regions in the world, namely Australia and New Zealand in the Southern hemisphere, and Canada and the U.S. in the Northern hemisphere. Table 9.1 shows the frequency and percentage distribution of Falun Gong and non–Falun Gong respondents living in these two regions.

Table 9.1 Country of residence – Falun Gong versus non–Falun Gong respondents

Country of residence	Falun Gong respondents		Non–Falun Gong respondents	
	Frequency	Percent	Frequency	Percent
Australia/NZ	154	43	151	66
Canada/US	114	32	35	15
Total	268	75	186	81

The figures could indicate that mainland Chinese and Asian-born Falun Gong respondents residing in these regions of the world were either individuals on temporary resident visas (for example, students, long-term visitors) or immigrants. This seems consistent with Falun Gong practitioners in North America being "a product of recent Chinese immigration" (Ownby, 2003b, p. 309; 2008a, p. 134).

Australia/New Zealand and Canada/United States appeared to be preferred destinations either for the pursuit of higher education or migration for many Falun Gong respondents. That there were more Australia-born and New

Zealand-born non–Falun Gong respondents could imply that many Falun Gong respondents residing in the countries they migrated to either did not have many non–Falun Gong mainland Chinese friends, or family members living outside of China, or they assimilated well and made more friends with people from other ethnic backgrounds.

Secondly, it could also imply that their non–Falun Gong mainland Chinese immigrant friends and relatives were fearful and negatively influenced by the CCP persecution of Falun Gong practitioners, and hence did not wish to participate in the survey. The fact that non–Falun Gong respondents accepted Falun Gong respondents' invitations to complete the online survey may have reflected their sincerity and receptiveness to Falun Gong, and/or support for their Falun Gong family/friends.

9.3.3 English as the first language

Nearly two-thirds of Falun Gong respondents (63%, n=226) reported that English was not their first language; 44% (n=164) reported Mandarin or a Chinese dialect as the language they grew up with. In contrast, more non–Falun Gong respondents (57%, n=130) reported English as their first language. This was reflected in the findings for country of birth, which indicated that there were more Falun Gong respondents born in mainland China and Asia where Mandarin and/or Chinese dialects were spoken, and with more non–Falun Gong respondents (40%) born in Australia and New Zealand.

9.3.4 Differences in medical history and health status

Findings showed distinct differences between Falun Gong and non–Falun Gong respondents in their reported medical and health conditions, the number of times they consulted a medical practitioner, their use of medications and health supplements, and in the amount of money they spent on medical and health expenses. Most Falun Gong respondents (88%, n=316) did not consult a medical practitioner; only 8.3% of Falun Gong respondents (n=30) visited a medical practitioner one to three times during the six-month period prior to completing this survey. Those who consulted a medical practitioner did so for minor health issues, a routine medical checkup, or work-related reasons such as procuring a medical certificate, whereas non–Falun Gong respondents identified more medical conditions and consulted medical practitioners more frequently.

Consistent with their self-reports of very low or no incidence of medical consultation, little or no use of medication and health supplements, 92% of Falun Gong respondents (n=330) did not spend any money on medical and health expenses. The eight percent of Falun Gong respondents (n=30) who reported medical and health expenditure had included government (Medicare payments for Australian residents) and private health insurance payments. The issue of Falun Gong practitioners not consulting a medical practitioner and not taking medications as often as non–Falun Gong individuals has often been misunderstood and misconstrued (Xie & Zhu, 2004). This controversy and allegations from the Chinese Communist regime were presented and discussed in *China and the future of Falun Gong* (Ownby, 2008a).

The teachings of Falun Gong do not prohibit medical treatment, medication intake or accessing medical care (Xie & Zhu, 2004). From the perspective of non–Falun Gong individuals, Falun Gong teachings seem to discourage practitioners from taking medicine or seeking medical treatment. However, this may not be that different from individuals living a naturalistic lifestyle who choose holistic health care approaches and refute conventional allopathic medical care because of their values and beliefs.

The health-wellness benefits and healing potential of Falun Gong can be some of the initial attractions to the practice. Findings from this research revealed that nearly one-third of Falun Gong respondents (31%, n=111) reported that besides Falun Gong teachings, spiritual elevation gained from the practice and other reasons, the prospect of physical and mental health benefits was what had first attracted them to Falun Gong. In addition, two Falun Gong respondents reported that they were searching for qigong or some form of exercise for health improvement. This finding was consistent with the results from previous studies (Ownby, 2008a; S. J. Palmer, 2003).

9.3.5 Differences in lifestyles between Falun Gong and non–Falun Gong respondents

Differences between Falun Gong and non–Falun Gong respondents were also reflected in their lifestyle habits such as cigarette smoking, alcohol consumption and recreational drug use. Falun Gong respondents were very healthy individuals with healthy lifestyle habits. Nearly all of them were non-cigarette smokers who did not drink alcohol or use recreational drugs. Two of the five Falun Gong respondents who reported smoking cigarettes were new practitioners who had been practicing Falun Gong for a period of six months to two years. Only eight Falun Gong respondents reported consuming alcohol and one Falun Gong respondent reported using recreational drugs.

Most Falun Gong respondents reported changing their lifestyle habits after commencing Falun Gong practice. When asked in Section 3 (Meditation Practice) of HW1 if they stopped smoking after starting Falun Gong practice, 82.3% (n=56) of those who smoked (n=68) stated that they quit their smoking habit after they began Falun Gong. Of those (n=174) who reported consuming alcohol, 97% (n=168) indicated they stopped after starting Falun Gong practice. Only six Falun Gong respondents did not give up alcohol consumption.

This lifestyle change could be explained from the Falun Gong perspective. The teachings of Falun Gong state that unhealthy lifestyles and addictions to substance use should be given up like attachments to be relinquished in order for a cultivator to make mind-body and spiritual improvements (H. Li, 2001b). Mr. Li Hongzhi, the founder and teacher of Falun Gong, explained that a Falun Gong practitioner's body has different forms of *gong* or cultivation energy and that drinking alcohol would diminish this cultivation energy and abilities (H. Li, 2001b). He stated that "it is quite loathsome if you become addicted to this habit, for drinking alcohol can make one irrational" (H. Li, 2001b, p. 279). Falun Gong practice cultivates the main consciousness (H. Li, 2001a, 2001b) and drinking alcohol causes the main consciousness to lose awareness and the ability to think rationally. Smoking is considered a strong desire, an attachment that "does not do the human body any good," and "if a person smokes for a long period of time, at the time of autopsy a doctor will find that his or her trachea and lungs are all black" (H. Li, 2001b, p. 280).

Since Falun Gong is a mind-body cultivation practice, it involves body purification:

> *Don't we practitioners want to purify our bodies? We should constantly purify our bodies and constantly progress toward high levels. Yet you still put that in your body, so aren't you going the opposite way from us? (H. Li, 2001b, p. 280).*

The absence of or lower alcohol consumption and smoking are reliable predictors of a better health-wellness outcome, according to Koenig (2004b; 2002) in discussing the link between psychoneuroimmunology (PNI), spirituality/religion and health. Spiritual/religious beliefs and spiritual practices were shown to foster positive and healthy behaviors, such as lower alcohol consumption and cigarette smoking, and discouraging unhealthy behaviors like drug use, risky sexual practices and other unsafe activities (Koenig, 2004b; Koenig & Cohen, 2002). Falun Gong respondents generally give up these addictive habits with the spiritual teachings to guide and sustain them. This is a likely and feasible explanation for the majority of Falun Gong respondents experiencing better health-wellness than non–Falun Gong respondents.

9.4 Findings from the SF-36 Health Survey

Falun Gong respondents consistently reported better health-wellness than non–Falun Gong respondents in the SF-36 Health Survey. Pearson chi-square results in Chapter 4 indicated that the differences between the two groups were statistically significant for all of the 36 items in the SF-36 Health Survey. A total of 88% of Falun Gong respondents (n=317) reported very good or excellent general health status, whereas only 53% of non–Falun Gong respondents (n=119) perceived their general health status as very good or excellent.

Falun Gong respondents experienced better health-wellness than non–Falun Gong respondents, suggesting that the practice of Falun Gong could have a positive health-wellness effect. Although no causal link could be verified from this research, the findings reflect the results of the health surveys conducted in mainland China (Author Unknown, 1998; Authors Unknown, 2002; Dan et al., 1998; Wang et al., 1998; Zhang & Xiao, 1996) and other Falun Gong health-wellness-related studies conducted outside of mainland China (Authors Unknown, 1999, 2003a; Lau, 2001; Q. Li et al., 2005; Lio et al., 2003).

There was a marked difference between Falun Gong and non–Falun Gong respondents in their self-perceived health. More than three-quarters of Falun Gong respondents (76%, n=274) perceived their health-wellness as excellent whereas only 19% of non–Falun Gong respondents (n=44) perceived themselves similarly. The majority of Falun Gong respondents (90%, n=324) reported, "Definitely false" to the statement, "I expect my health to get worse," whereas only about a third of non–Falun Gong respondents (37%, n=84) disagreed with the same statement. Similarly, 87% of Falun Gong respondents (n=313) disagreed with the statement, "I seem to get sick a little easier than other people" compared to 47% of non–Falun Gong respondents (n=108).

Findings also revealed that Falun Gong respondents reported more health problems than non–Falun Gong respondents prior to commencing Falun Gong practice. Forty-five percent of Falun Gong respondents (n=163) specified medical conditions they had prior to Falun Gong practice, with 50% of them reporting two or more medical conditions. Findings from this research indicated that since taking up Falun Gong practice, many reported they perceived a significant improvement in their medical and health conditions, suggesting that the practice of Falun Gong could have a positive health-wellness effect.

The literature review in Chapter 2 included the power of the mind, the importance of positive thinking and positive emotions, that "matter and mind are one thing" (H. Li, 2001b, p. 28), and that the mind can influence health and wellness. The teachings of Falun Gong in *Zhuan Falun* state:

> *As a practitioner, if you always think that it is an illness, you are actually asking for it. If you ask for an illness, it will come inside your body. As a practitioner, your xinxing level should be high. You should not always worry that it is an illness, for this fear of illness is an attachment and it can bring you trouble just the same (H. Li, 2001b, p. 218).*

The review also discussed the strong and positive link between spirituality/religion and health. That Falun Gong respondents perceived themselves to have and reported having excellent health-wellness status could be explained by their involvement and spiritual commitment to Falun Gong practice. Falun Gong respondents were more optimistic and had more positive self-perception about their current and future health-wellness status than non–Falun Gong respondents. Having strong positive and righteous thoughts is an important and necessary aspect in Falun Gong practice. Hence one of the three essential responsibilities of Falun Gong practitioners is 'sending forth righteous thoughts' (SFRT), a 15-minute special meditation that is practiced four times daily to help clear and eliminate negative thoughts, all kinds of negativity and undesirable elements (Clearwisdom editors, 2004; H. Li, 2002). Having righteous thoughts is fundamental in Falun Gong: "So, as you go about cultivation, you must cultivate your mind, get rid of human attachments, and view things with righteous thoughts" (H. Li, 2008, p. 4).

The concept of having righteous thoughts, positive thinking and optimism, a vital quality in Falun Gong cultivation practice, and its health-wellness effects is not new. In the science of happiness or mind-body happiness, researchers such as Martin Seligman, former president of the American Psychological Association (APA), considered optimism as a health-wellness promoting quality linked with "good physical health, less depression and mental illness, longer life and, yes, greater happiness" (cited in Wallis, 2005, p. 44). The literature review in Chapter 2 discussed the importance of having positive states of mind and emotions such as hope, joy, tranquility, optimism, positive thinking and righteous thoughts, and how these qualities foster better health and wellness outcomes. Thus maintaining righteous thoughts, having positive thinking, optimism, and other positive emotions can have a powerful effect on a person's health and wellness (Fredrickson, 2000; Lemonick, 2005; H. Li, 2001b; Wallis, 2005), whereas negative emotions such as anger, anxiety, envy, fear, and jealousy have detrimental effects on a person's physiology and state of mind (Maciocia, 1989). Traditional Chinese medicine recognizes that negative emotions affect internal organs, the immune, nervous and endocrine systems, and other bodily functions (Maciocia, 1989), causing imbalances and various illnesses. The effects of negative emotions are expressed in these words:

> *Therefore, he competes and fights all his life with a badly wounded heart. He might feel very bitter and tired, always finding things unfair. Being unable to eat or sleep well, he feels sad and disappointed. When he gets*

older, he will end up in poor health and all kinds of illnesses will surface
(H. Li, 2001b, pp. 284-285).

Practicing Falun Gong reinforces positive qualities or states of mind as practitioners strive to follow the teachings of Falun Gong to their best ability, without pursuit for fame, gain or health-wellness benefits. Falun Gong teaches practicing *wuwei* in speech, thoughts and actions, which means taking the path of non-action, without intention (H. Li, 2001b) or pursuit. In letting go of pursuit, the mind is liberated to "simultaneous cultivation of Zhen, Shan, and Ren" (H. Li, 2001a, p. 61) and adherence to the principles of truthfulness, compassion and forbearance. Besides practicing to maintain the state of *wuwei* in daily life, this state can be achieved through meditation—sitting in the state of *ding*: "When one practices in this state, the body is being fully transformed, and it is the optimum state" (H. Li, 2001b, p. 339). When this optimum state manifests, the mind-body and spirit become integrated and true healing can take place; this can have health-wellness benefits for Falun Gong practitioners.

9.5 How Falun Gong can lead to better health and wellness

Findings indicated that Falun Gong had transformed the lives of Falun Gong respondents in the following aspects: changes in physical, mental and emotional health; stress coping ability; relationships with significant others; and attitude towards life. Table 9.2 shows a summary of perceived significant improvements across these health-wellness aspects.

Table 9.2 Summary of perceived significant improvement since Falun Gong practice

Change since practicing Falun Gong	Significantly Improved	
	Frequency	Percent
Change in physical health	297	82.5
Change in mental and emotional health	325	90.3
Change in stress coping ability	317	88.1
Change in relationship with significant others	252	70.0
Change in attitude to life	335	93.1

These perceived improvements in multi-dimensions of health-wellness for Falun Gong respondents are consistent with other health surveys conducted in mainland China (Author Unknown, 1998; Authors Unknown, 2002; Dan et al., 1998; Wang et al., 1998; Zhang & Xiao, 1996) and outside of China (Authors Unknown, 1999, 2003a; Lau, 2001; Q. Li et al., 2005; Lio et al., 2003).

The majority of Falun Gong respondents (91%, n=328) revealed that the secret to their health and wellness was "improving xinxing or moral character," while 78% (n=280) attributed it to "regular study of Falun Gong teachings." Falun Gong exercise routine followed this (47%, n=170), with 44% of respondents (n=158) stating that a positive change of attitude towards life, that is, having righteous, positive thoughts and being optimistic, was also an important factor in the Falun Gong health-wellness equation.

Improving *xinxing,* or upgrading moral character and following the principles of truthfulness, compassion and forbearance (Zhen-Shan-Ren) is considered the core of Falun Gong practice (H. Li, 2001b). Every Falun Gong practitioner aspires to embody these teachings in their daily life. Regular study of Falun Gong teachings and SFRT special meditation to maintain positive and righteous thoughts are two important aspects of Falun Gong practice. Being true, good and enduring, as embodied in the Falun Gong truthfulness, compassion, and forbearance (Zhen-Shan-Ren) principles, is not a New Age spiritual fad. These are universal moral principles taught by all major religious, philosophical and spiritual teachings. Being good and doing good has its roots in both ancient Eastern traditions (such as Taoism and Confucianism) and Western traditions (as in Christianity). Aristotle, the Greek philosopher, expounded that attaining true happiness or wellbeing involved virtue or goodness, as in having good moral behavior and sound reasoning based on wisdom (Easton, 2005).

Respondent 196 stated that what had led to their better health and wellness was the "body purification by *Shifu*" (Chinese term for Master). Mr. Li Hongzhi did not claim that Falun Gong was a cure for illnesses (Xie & Zhu, 2004), although he initially did participate in healing activities to support a CCP-organized qigong exhibition (H. Li, 2001b). He succinctly explained that body purification was part of the cultivation process:

I do not talk about healing illness here, nor will we heal illness. As a genuine practitioner, however, you cannot practice cultivation with an ill body. I will purify your body. The body purification will be done only for those who come to truly learn the practice and the Fa (H. Li, 2001b, p. 3).

We will purify their bodies and enable them to practice cultivation toward high levels. There is a transition at the lowest level of cultivation practice, and this is to purify your body completely. All the bad things on your mind, the karmic field surrounding your body, and the elements that make your body unhealthy will be cleaned out. If they are not cleaned out, how could you, with such an impure, dark body and a filthy mind, practice cultivation towards a higher level? (H. Li, 2001b, p. 6).

Certainly, the bad things in your body, including illnesses, must be removed first, but we do not treat illness here. We are purifying your body, and the term is not "healing illness," either. We just call it "purifying the body," and we clean out the bodies of true practitioners (H. Li, 2001b, p. 40).

This body purification is no different from the detoxification process or healing reactions from CAM or MBM holistic intervention therapies (Wilson, 2011). Some Falun Gong individuals experienced vomiting, diarrhea, nasal mucus discharge, flu-like symptoms, discharging of pus or blood in their excrement, or showing symptoms of previously cured illnesses, shortly after starting Falun Gong practice (H. Li, 2001b) before feeling better. The literature review in Chapter 2 discussed these physical and emotional healing reactions as side effects and adverse effects of meditation. In contrast, Dr. Wilson (2011) stated that these healing reactions are "welcome signs of healing" (p. 1), necessary for true healing to take place and not to be mistaken for illness symptoms or worsening of a health condition.

To gain insight into how Falun Gong leads to better health and wellness, it is necessary to discuss some of the Falun Gong concepts within the context of Falun Gong cultivation practice. The first is the cultivation of *xinxing* or improvement of one's moral character and conduct. The majority of Falun Gong respondents (91%, n=328) reported that improving *xinxing* led to better health and wellness. *Xinxing* is explained as follows:

It includes de (a type of matter), tolerance, enlightenment quality, sacrifice, giving up ordinary people's different desires and attachments, being able to suffer hardships, and so on. It encompasses various things. Every aspect of xinxing must be upgraded for you to make real progress (H. Li, 2001b, p. 28).

Xinxing cultivation refers to cultivating the heart and mind, being calm and compassionate, caring less about personal feelings and desires, and not vying for personal gain or self-validation in a conflict with others. The aim of cultivation is to aspire to a much higher standard of moral conduct in everyday life:

You should always maintain a heart of compassion and kindness. ... You should always be benevolent and kind to others, and consider others when doing anything. ... you should first consider whether others can put up with this matter or if it will hurt anyone (2001b, p. 162).

Throughout *Zhuan Falun* (H. Li, 2001b), Falun Gong practitioners are reminded that "True cultivation practice depends fully upon your heart" (p. 92), that "without cultivating the heart, no one can make it" (p. 102), and hence "you must truly cultivate your heart to make it work" (p. 102). Thus a change of heart or tempering of the heart is essential in Falun Gong cultivation practice, just as a change of thoughts from negative thoughts to positive, righteous thoughts is required in Falun Gong cultivation by doing regular SFRT meditation to clear the negative energy field.

Karma, the law of cause and effect is also of relevance (H. Li, 2001a, 2001b). According to Falun Gong teachings, every illness condition has a corresponding dark or black energy field caused by karma (H. Li, 2001a, 2001b). To truly heal an illness, this karmic energy field needs to be eliminated and replaced with a positive energy field or *de. De,* translated as "virtue," is a pure white energy field, that envelopes a person and is required for *xinxing*, heart-mind improvement and spiritual elevation (H. Li, 2001b).

Virtue is acquired through undergoing hardships, trials and tribulations in everyday life (H. Li, 2001b). The karma elimination and transformation process is explained here:

From today on, some people will feel chilly all over their bodies as though they suffer a heavy cold, and their bones may ache as well. Most of you will feel uncomfortable somewhere. Your legs may ache and your head may feel dizzy. The ill part of your body, which you thought was healed before through qigong exercises or by a qigong master, will again have illness. ... We must dig it out and eliminate it completely from its root. With this, you may feel that your illnesses have recurred. This is to remove your karma fundamentally. Thus you will have reactions. Some people may have physical reactions somewhere. Some may feel uncomfortable in one way or another, as different kinds of discomfort will manifest. These are all normal. ... When you feel very uncomfortable, it indicates that things will turn around after reaching the extreme point. Your whole body will be purified and it must be completely purified (H. Li, 2001b, p. 89).

Falun Gong practitioners will go through body purification, cleansing, elimination, and transformation of the illness karma during cultivation practice, thereby resulting in better health and wellness. The concepts of illness karma and the body purification process provide insights into why so few Falun Gong respondents consult a medical practitioner, take medication and herbal supplements, and why the majority of them experience better health-wellness than non–Falun Gong respondents.

Falun Gong teaches that the primary purpose of being a human being is to "return to one's origin and true self" (H. Li, 2001b, p. 5) through cultivation. This process entails relinquishing all psychological and behavioral attachments, desires, and addictions such as smoking, alcohol consumption, drug use, gambling, and other vices. For the sake of cultivation and the genuine wish to gain spiritual elevation and return to one's original true self, practitioners are motivated to modify their behaviors and integrate the teachings of Falun Gong into their daily life. In other words, Falun Gong practitioners strive to be "true, good, and endure" (H. Li, 2003, pp. 12, 13) for delayed gratification—the wish to return to one's original true self one day—with health and wellness as the immediate by-product of their current cultivation state. Findings from this research suggest that Falun Gong helps to elicit beneficial behavior modification, perceived improvements in physical, mental and emotional health, stress-coping ability, relationships with significant others, a positive change of attitude towards life, and an optimistic perception of the current and future health-wellness status of those individuals who genuinely embrace Falun Gong practice.

Besides the heart-mind cultivation, Falun Gong exercises help to enhance health, healing, and wellness by opening up hundreds of energy channels in the human body, increasing energy flow, purifying the body of toxins, and rectifying all energy blockages in the body (H. Li, 2001a). In the discourse on the "Heaven Circuit" in Lecture 8 of *Zhuan Falun* (H. Li, 2001b, pp. 323-337), Falun Gong practice is explained as enabling the simultaneous opening of these numerous energy channels until they eventually merge into one large energy pathway. According to traditional Chinese medicine, ill health and disease stem from the obstruction of energy channels, causing deficiency or stagnation of *qi* and blood (Maciocia, 1989). Optimum mind-body, spiritual health and wellness, and the prevention of illness can be achieved and maintained when the energy channels widen and merge into one. In Falun Gong, when this point is reached, the cultivator has reached the highest form of "In-Triple-World-Fa (Shi-Jian-Fa) cultivation" (H. Li, 2001b, pp. 6, 336), the first of the two major levels of cultivation practice (H. Li, 2001b). At this level, the high-energy matter will transform the human body: "one's body will be white and pure, the skin will be fair and delicate" (H. Li, 2001b, p. 336). Understanding this concept and other fundamental teachings of Falun Gong will provide a deeper insight into Falun Gong respondents' motivation and diligence in their cultivation practice and how Falun Gong has health-wellness enhancing benefits, as the findings of this research have indicated.

Most Falun Gong respondents in this research were veteran practitioners with a sound understanding of Falun Gong teachings. Over half of the Falun Gong respondents (54%, n=194) had been practicing Falun Gong from six to more than ten years, and less than 10% (n=35) reported practicing Falun Gong for less than two years. Most Falun Gong respondents were diligent with their Falun Gong exercise routine; more than half of the respondents (58%, n=203) engaged in daily practice or four to five times a week. Nearly three-quarters of Falun Gong respondents (72%, n=253) engaged in daily Fa study and almost all Falun Gong respondents (99%, n=349) spent some time each week on Fa study. That these dedicated Falun Gong respondents did not consult medical practitioners, used little or no medication, and experienced very good to excellent health-wellness status could be because they are experienced meditators who had practiced Falun Gong for a number of years. The literature review in Chapter 2 indicated a difference in the therapeutic effects of meditation between novice and experienced meditators (Goldberg, 1982).

Another crucial aspect of Falun Gong cultivation is the requirement for practitioners to honestly look within, examine themselves, identify, and get rid of their attachments. It can be said that Falun Gong enhances mind-body awareness, awareness of self and especially of others, and it influences self-motivation to be true, good, and endure. Falun Gong teachings enable practitioners to approach life's challenges differently; hence their propensity for physical and mental illness is reduced and the person's health-wellness status improves or is maintained, as the findings from this research have indicated. Likewise, the strong sense of belief, faith, and discipline in the cultivation practice contribute to homeostasis, equanimity, and the practitioner's health-wellness.

For the sake of cultivation and genuinely wishing to gain spiritual elevation and return to one's original true self, veteran Falun Gong respondents are motivated to modify their behaviors and integrate Falun Gong teachings into their daily life. Falun Gong teachings offer practical guidance for daily living, conforming maximally and living in everyday society, with a family, a job, house, car, and other material possessions, like non–Falun Gong individuals. Falun Gong respondents are artists, business/computer information technology professionals, counselors, doctors, educators, journalists, scientists, students, and people of all ages, ethnicities, and nationalities, as indicated in the findings. Besides their better health-wellness status, Falun Gong respondents are no different from non–Falun Gong respondents and other citizens in society.

Findings from this research suggest that the key to the health-wellness effects of Falun Gong lies in four important aspects of the practice: heart-mind or *xinxing* cultivation; study of the teachings; practice of the exercises; and having positive and righteous thoughts. However, no causal link between Falun Gong/spirituality and health-wellness can be established from this research. This is an area open for future Falun Gong studies. Nonetheless, there is something inherent in Falun Gong, indiscernible to human logic, that seems to work wonders for these veteran Falun Gong respondents when they maintain all the core aspects of cultivation. Findings show that many Falun Gong respondents experience perceived significant improvements in the different health-wellness domains, suggesting that Falun Gong could be an ideal alternative mind-body spiritual cultivation practice for people from all walks of life—the young, the busy professional, and older people seeking overall improvement of mind, body, and spirit.

9.6 Reporting of adverse findings

To maintain transparency and research credibility, it is relevant to report adverse findings from this research. Results indicating Falun Gong practice had worsened health conditions or had no difference were very low, as shown in Table 9.3.

Table 9.3 Summary of worsening of conditions since Falun Gong practice

Change since practicing Falun Gong across five health-wellness dimensions	Significantly worse		Slightly worse		No difference	
	Frequency	%	Frequency	%	Frequency	%
Change in physical health	1	0.3	1	0.3	5	1.4
Change in mental & emotional health	1	0.3	1	0.3	1	0.3
Change in stress coping ability	1	0.3	1	0.3	3	0.8
Change in relationship with significant others	1	0.3	7	1.9	16	4.4
Change in attitude to life	1	0.3	1	0.3	1	0.3

In fact, the same Falun Gong respondent (R27) reported a significant worsening of their medical condition across all five health-wellness dimensions. Respondent 27 was a veteran Falun Gong practitioner with a good understanding of Falun Gong and had practiced Falun Gong for four to six years, engaging in exercise practice two to three times a week, and daily Fa study, 11 to 15 hours a week.

There could be different reasons why a small number of Falun Gong respondents experienced significant, slight worsening, or no difference in the above-mentioned five health-wellness dimensions. The number of years of Falun Gong practice, frequency of exercise practice and Fa study, or time spent on practice and Fa study could explain worsening or absence of change in health status.

The worsening of conditions since commencing Falun Gong practice had not deterred this respondent, who acknowledged practicing Falun Gong not for health benefits but due to "a predestined relationship." It would be a strong belief in predestined relationship (yuanfen) and faith in Falun Gong to continue with the practice despite the worsening of their condition across all five health-wellness dimensions. It needs to be stressed that the ultimate goal of Falun Gong cultivation is not for healing and fitness, but for spiritual enlightenment and to return to one's origin and true self (H. Li, 2001b). Falun Gong is not a panacea, but a strong precursor for mental health prowess, better health-wellness and overall mind-body and spiritual improvement.

In CAM and MBM therapies, healing and purification reactions, or a reversal process may arise where past health conditions or symptoms reappear before the person gets better (Wilson, 2011). Wilson (2011) explained the difference between healing and illness symptoms—the former is often mild, passes quickly and is peculiar in that one may have a sore throat, fever or flu symptoms without feeling tired. Like CAM or MBM therapies, Falun Gong practice has contraindications. Mr. Li stated that people with serious illnesses should seek medical treatment because Falun Gong practice is not for healing illnesses (H. Li, 2001b). Because Falun Gong cultivates the main consciousness, it is not suitable for those with mental illness such as psychosis (H. Li, 2001b) and other serious psychiatric disorders, such as schizophrenia or mania characterized by delusions, hallucinations, incoherence, and distortions in perceptions of reality.

9.7 Summary

This concludes Chapter 9, which has presented a discussion of the findings from this research and provided insights into the potential for Falun Gong to maintain and enhance health and wellness. Readers must bear in mind that this discussion is based on the findings of this research and that greater knowledge of and insight into Falun Gong can only be obtained through reading the teachings of Falun Gong.

Falun Gong has been shown to be a beneficial mind-body Eastern spiritual cultivation practice with potential use in counseling and health-wellness promotion for people of all ages and from all walks of life. The practice has led to better health and wellness experiences for Falun Gong respondents. Apart from their better health-wellness status, attributed to Falun Gong practice, Falun Gong respondents are no different from non–Falun Gong respondents and other citizens in society. It can be said that the key to the health-wellness effects of Falun Gong lies in maintaining the key aspects of the practice: heart-mind or *xinxing* cultivation, study of teachings and practice of the exercises, and having positive and righteous thoughts.

Chapter 10, the concluding chapter, will address the limitations and strengths of this research, recommendations for future studies, the role of Falun Gong as a counseling adjunct, and recommendations for counselors and other health professionals on how to assist and work with Falun Gong practitioners.

CHAPTER 10

Conclusion

Sometimes the best things in life are free. (Oz, 2003, p. 2)

10.1 Chapter overview

This concluding chapter presents a chapter synopsis and an overall summary of this research. It discusses the limitations and strengths of this research and offers both Falun Gong and non–Falun Gong readers, including researchers, counselors and other health professionals, practical recommendations and resources relating to future studies on Falun Gong, the use and integration of Falun Gong in counseling practices and other health services, and in health-wellness promotion.

This research comprised two parts. The aims of Part A were to obtain an international demographic profile of Falun Gong respondents and to ascertain any possible differences or similarities between Falun Gong and non–Falun Gong respondents in terms of their demographic profile. The aims of Part B of this research were to investigate the health-wellness effects of Falun Gong as perceived by Falun Gong practitioners; and to determine whether individuals who practice Falun Gong experience better health-wellness status than those who do not.

Chapter 1 gave an overview of this dissertation and provided an introduction to Falun Gong, the aims, scope of this research, and definitions of related terms and key concepts. It introduced the positive link between spirituality/religion and health, which forms the theoretical framework for this research. Chapter 2 presented a comprehensive general literature review and critical analysis of studies and literature relating to the effects of meditation. It provided the historical contexts, trends in meditative practices, roles and effects of meditation (in the helping professions). Chapter 3 focused on a Falun Gong-related literature review, existing studies on Falun Gong, and literature exploring the positive link between spirituality/religion and health. Chapter 4 described the research design, approach and methodology, as well as the three main phases of the research. It explained the rationale for the choice of a descriptive cross-sectional online survey using a mixed methods approach and the use of self-report questionnaires.

Chapter 5 presented the findings for Falun Gong respondents for the two parts of this research, while Chapter 6 reported the findings from the non–Falun Gong respondents. Data was reported and analyzed using mostly descriptive statistics with Pearson chi-square tests, and presented according to the order of the items in the surveys. Chapter 7 was dedicated to the written comments from both Falun Gong and non–Falun Gong respondents. Chapter 8 involved a comparison between the two groups of respondents.

Chapter 9 provided an analysis and discussion of the findings and provided insight into Falun Gong practitioners and the health-wellness effects of Falun Gong. The chapter also explained what the findings meant in terms of Falun Gong, why Falun Gong works, and how Falun Gong has led to better health-wellness experiences in individuals who practice it. The discussion provided some understanding of Falun Gong as a beneficial mind-body Eastern meditative movement and spiritual cultivation practice with potential use in counseling and health-wellness promotion.

Chapter 10 comprises the final chapter of the doctoral dissertation and presents an overall view of the chapters in the dissertation. It discusses the limitations and strengths of this research and offers practical recommendations for both Falun Gong and non–Falun Gong readers, including researchers, counselors, and other health professionals. It includes some resources relating to future studies on Falun Gong, the use and integration of Falun Gong in counseling practices, and other health services, as well as suggestions for health-wellness promotion.

10.2 Synopsis and significance of findings

This research has achieved the aims of both parts of the research. Findings for Part A have provided a snapshot of the demographic profile of Falun Gong respondents around the world. More than half the Falun Gong respondents (54%, n=194) are experienced and long-term practitioners who reported practicing Falun Gong for six to 10 years. About 60% of them are female, most of them married, with tertiary education qualifications and professional careers. Thirty percent of Falun Gong respondents (n=107) have a master's, PhD, or doctoral degree. The average age of Falun Gong respondents around the world (outside of mainland China) is in the 30 to 39 years age and 40 to 49 years age range.

Findings for Part A highlighted similar demographic features between Falun Gong and non–Falun Gong respondents. The non–Falun Gong respondents also consisted mainly of females, from diverse ethnic backgrounds, married, with tertiary qualifications and professional careers. Falun Gong respondents were like non–Falun Gong respondents, married with families and similar occupations in society, like other citizens, with the exception of their spiritual beliefs and Falun Gong practice that offers them health-wellness benefits.

Findings for Part B suggested that Falun Gong has positive health-wellness effects on Falun Gong practitioners, and those individuals who practice Falun Gong experience better health and wellness than those who do not. Falun Gong respondents reported being very healthy, with healthy lifestyle habits. Nearly all were non-smokers who did not consume alcohol or take recreational drugs, which are reasonable indicators and predictors of a better health-wellness status. Since commencing Falun Gong practice, they rarely visit medical practitioners, take any medications, or spend money on medical and health expenses. Observed health-wellness differences between Falun Gong and non–Falun Gong respondents have been shown in this research. Falun Gong respondents are more likely to report excellent health, no or little use of medication, and hardly any medical or health expenses compared to non–Falun Gong respondents. Findings for Part B indicated that people who practice Falun Gong have more positive and optimistic perceptions of their health-wellness status.

Findings depicted a demographic profile of young, educated and career-oriented individuals from diverse ethnic backgrounds who are drawn to the teachings of Falun Gong. Demographically, Falun Gong respondents do not appear to be different or unlike non–Falun Gong respondents. The majority of Falun Gong respondents work for a living; only 2.5% of Falun Gong respondents (n=9) are unemployed. They have families and occupations. They pay tax and contribute to the society they live in as do non–Falun Gong respondents. These Falun Gong respondents are certainly not a group of ignorant people deluded by a spiritual meditation practice banned by the Chinese Communist Party (CCP), much as the CCP would like the rest of the world to think and believe.

Findings suggested that their spiritual beliefs and practice offer them optimum health-wellness benefits. Although no causal links can be derived from the findings, the literature review has indicated that there is a positive link between spirituality/religion and health. This could be the underlying reason why more Falun Gong respondents reported excellent health and more positive perceptions of their health-wellness status than non–Falun Gong respondents. Falun Gong teachings affirm that "it's known that what actually causes people to become ill is seventy percent psychological and thirty percent physiological" (H. Li, 2001b, p. 218), and that "matter and mind are one thing" (H. Li, 2001b, p. 28). Ninety-two per cent of Falun Gong respondents (n=329) perceived the study of Falun Gong teachings to be the most important in their practice. These respondents indicated practicing Falun Gong exercises and studying the teachings regularly. They reported experiencing perceived significant improvements in their physical, mental and emotional health since practicing Falun Gong. They had a positive perception of their health and constantly focused on having positive, righteous thoughts. Most importantly, they believe and have faith in their spiritual practice.

The findings support Falun Gong as a beneficial mind-body health-wellness meditative movement and spiritual cultivation practice that may have public medical and health care implications across society. Findings from this research support the power of the mind-body connection and the potential of Falun Gong as a preventative, mind-body and holistic bio-psycho-spiritual health-wellness lifestyle or a total mind-body-spirit healthcare system.

This research is noteworthy because of its process and significance as the first Australian-based Falun Gong research. Because of its international demographic profile and the uniqueness of the comparison of Falun Gong respondents with non–Falun Gong respondents, this research offers new insights into, and informed understanding of, Falun Gong. Readers, especially counseling and other health professionals, are encouraged to consider integrating Falun Gong into their work and everyday life for better health-wellness outcomes for themselves and their clients. They are invited to see the parallel between Falun Gong principles of truthfulness, compassion, and forbearance and the three core principles of the person-centered counseling approach (PCA)—unconditional positive regard, empathy, and congruence (Elliott & Freire, 2007; Mearns & Thorne, 2007; C. R. Rogers, 1951, 1957). This analogy can also offer guidance for best practice, understanding, and insight into the provision of quality help for Falun Gong individuals.

An outcome from this research is a six-step process that can be used in identifying and eliminating issues. The six-step process (see Table 10.1) can be a practical resource as a self-help tool or an intervention strategy that health professionals can integrate into their work with both Falun Gong and non–Falun Gong clients.

10.3 Limitations

The findings of this research should be considered within the context of its limitations. Despite the meticulous care and consideration given to the choice of design and methodology, the self-designed questionnaires, implementation of the surveys, data processing and data analysis, this research has several limitations.

The first limitation concerns the selection bias of non–Falun Gong respondents that comprised family members, friends or colleagues of Falun Gong respondents. They were invited or 'recruited' by Falun Gong respondents who might have been biased in the invitation process and may have chosen the least healthy or least well non–Falun Gong family member or friend to complete the survey. This is, however, beyond the control of the researcher. As discussed in Chapter 4 there is no one 'correct' process as long as the researcher is aware and understands the pros and cons relating to the choice of the comparison group. It is pertinent to consider, however, that Falun Gong teachings indicate that the health-wellness status of non–Falun Gong family members living in close proximity with Falun Gong individuals may also improve (H. Li, 2001b), and this could influence the data and reduce the contrast between the two groups. Several Falun Gong respondents also expressed this via emails to the researcher.

> I also got my husband (a non-practitioner) to complete the survey... I realized that as my husband was completing the survey, his answers to the questions were not that dissimilar to mine (as a practitioner), even though he is a smoker and drinks alcohol. I then realized that his results on the survey may reflect the fact that he lives with a practitioner, as in the past he was quite a sickly person but over the past couple of years he has been quite good.

> Just wanted to mention this, that an everyday [non–Falun Gong] person's health can be improved by living with a practitioner and I'm not sure whether you had taken this into account in your survey. I wonder how many other practitioners will get their family members to complete the survey, thinking that they are everyday people when in fact potentially there could be some bias there from living with a practitioner [30 July 2007].

> As I see it, that can complicate your survey, if you are measuring the difference between practitioners and non-practitioners and if the non-practitioners can be recruited from family and friends. One can be in very close contact to one's spouse for a considerable percentage of time. The practitioner's spouse would then benefit from the practitioner, which would interfere with what you are trying to establish. It would lessen the contrast in benefits [31 July 2007].

However, this possibility did not appear to influence the findings. Despite the observed similarities in demographic profile between non–Falun Gong and Falun Gong respondents, the differences in their reports for the SF-36 Health Survey were further verified by the Pearson chi-square tests as statistically significant.

The second limitation involves the reliance on self-reports and self-assessment. As mentioned in Chapter 3, the researcher was aware of the limitations of self-report measures. One of the drawbacks is the susceptibility of self-reports to result in conscious or unconscious misrepresentation by respondents. The skeptic might contend that, since Falun Gong respondents were aware that the aim of this research was to investigate health-wellness effects of Falun Gong, their responses to the survey questions might reflect a bias to make themselves and Falun Gong look good. Nonetheless, self-reporting is a prevalent way of gathering information and collecting data in counseling research. Self-reports involve respondents assessing themselves on the premise that they answer the items honestly. Respondents' self-reports and perceptions of their health were important, relevant and valid. The researcher adopted the Rogerian person-centered "the client knows best" (Mearns & Thorne, 2007, p. 1) stance and trusted Falun Gong respondents to take righteous actions and adhere to the Falun Gong principles of truthfulness, compassion and forbearance. Another drawback of self-reports is that, unlike longitudinal studies, the data from this cross-sectional research was collected at the same time and hence no causal conclusions could be established. But it was not the aim of this research to prove a causal link between Falun Gong and health-wellness.

The third limitation relates to the use of the anonymous Internet-based survey. Because there was no face-to-face contact with respondents, the researcher could not validate the authenticity of their reports or whether respondents were genuinely Falun Gong practitioners and their family members or friends. Technical and Internet access glitches such as a browser freeze, server crash, and double entry could happen when respondents tried to complete the online survey. The online survey could limit respondents to those with computer skills, and computer and Internet access. In addition, because the online survey was in English, it may draw those proficient in that language to complete the survey, although Chinese translations of the HW1 and HW2 were posted on the website as a reference guide. The issue of whether or not the sample is representative of the target group may also arise. Other concerns included Internet security, possible interceptions of online survey responses and database hacking, which were beyond the control of the researcher, although steps were taken to manage the risks. However, given all of these potential issues, the use of the Internet was efficient and cost-effective, and the use of the online surveys did not seem to present any of the issues that were possible.

The fourth limitation concerns the self-designed questionnaire sections, specifically questions on ethnicity, income, medical and health expenses. No prescriptive range or options were provided for these questions making it a challenge to classify and especially to convert local currency to Australian currency. Perhaps a range of options could have been provided, including an "Other" category and another question asking respondents to specify what they mean by "Other" to address this.

Likewise, medical health insurance expenses could have been addressed as a separate question to avoid random reporting of private or government medical health insurance payments included as a medical and health expense. It was unclear if those who did report medical and health expenses included private and/or public health insurance payments. Most Australian respondents did not specifically report their compulsory Medicare (public health insurance program) payments because the contribution is automatically deducted from their gross income. One retired non–Falun Gong respondent (R39) who reported spending 30 Australian dollars explained, "Because I am a pensioner, I get medicines at concessions rate, like $3.80 per prescription." While the majority of Falun Gong respondents did not report any medical and health expenses, one Australian Falun Gong respondent (R222) reported spending AU$1,000 on gym membership and one Canadian Falun Gong respondent (R228) reported spending CA$400 on dental services. To capture this, an item could have been added asking for other medical and/or health-related expenses.

Finally, research bias can be another limitation that all research studies are susceptible to. To minimize research bias, the researcher endeavored to remain transparent throughout the entire research process. Conscious attempts were made at the onset in the choice of methodology and design. Other endeavors to reduce bias included using the online survey method, liaising only with members of the Falun Dafa associations, key regional contact persons or the pilot study members, maintaining distance from potential respondents during the data collection period to reduce the researcher's influence on respondents, and adopting an objective stance in the analysis and reporting of the findings. As well as this, the researcher held to the ethics requirements of the research and endeavored to emulate the Falun Gong qualities of truthfulness, compassion, and forbearance throughout the entire research and dissertation writing process.

10.4 Strengths

Despite the limitations, this research has several strengths, which include
the following:
- This Falun Gong research is Australian-based;
- It has an international focus;
- Efforts were made to match Falun Gong with non–Falun Gong respondents to reduce variability;
- It uses a mixed methods research approach;
- There were additional endeavors to minimize or eliminate researcher bias;
- A pilot study was conducted for research integrity;
- It uses technology to benefit the research process; and
- It includes reporting of all findings, including adverse, for authenticity.

This is an Australian-based health-wellness Falun Gong research project and
also the first with an international focus. Both Falun Gong and non–Falun
Gong respondents were from all over the world and from diverse ethnic and
cultural backgrounds. Efforts were made to match the two groups based on the
inclusion and exclusion criteria outlined in Table 4.1 and Table 4.2 in Chapter
4 on research design. Sample size was 360 for Falun Gong respondents and
230 for non-Falun Gong respondents. Despite the discrepancy in numbers
between the two groups, this did not influence the findings.

The choice of a mixed methods approach, frequently used in counseling
psychology and social sciences research, could also be considered another
strength. This method was chosen to broaden the scope, provide deeper
insights and enhance the analytical power of the research. Throughout the
entire research process, conscious attempts were made to minimize or eliminate
research bias to maintain credibility, consistency and reliability, which are the
characteristics of sound research (O'Leary, 2004). The researcher is aware that
findings are based solely on the self-reports and perceptions of respondents,
which may not necessarily represent or truly reflect the cultivation practice
and personal experience of Falun Gong practitioners in general. Nonetheless,
the findings are indicative and positive, well corroborated, and justify the
aims of this research.

Particular care was taken to be transparent and objective throughout the entire research process. This was to minimize or eliminate researcher bias and any possible influence from the personal experience and expectations of the researcher, based on the results from existing Falun Gong studies, and the positive reviews of studies examining the effects of other similar meditative movement practices, such as tai chi, qigong, yoga, and meditation. Care was also taken to be consistently authentic to the reports of the respondents and in the analysis, reporting, and presentation of the findings. The researcher wishes to emphasize that this research is not sponsored or funded by any Falun Dafa associations, or any Falun Gong individual, or organization. The request for Falun Dafa associations to place the URL web links of the surveys on the Falun Gong websites, and obtaining written approval from the Falun Dafa associations before commencing the research, were recommendations from the University's Human Research Ethics Committee during the ethics approval process, as explained in Chapter 3. This research was initiated and inspired by the researcher's interest in the possible integration of Falun Gong into professional counseling practice, combined with previous Falun Gong health and wellness projects that involved offering Falun Gong classes in community settings for counseling clients to attend.

An obvious strength of this research was the international pilot study process during the initial phase to obtain feedback on the self-designed questionnaire for HW1 and HW2 before the actual online survey commenced. The pilot study achieved its purpose well in the research process with beneficial feedback and recommendations. Pilot study members facilitated a vital communication link between the researcher and Falun Gong respondents during the data collection phase.

Another strength is the Internet administration of the survey, which minimized social desirability effects and fostered respondents' honesty and candor. Finally, the reporting of adverse findings reflects the researcher's consistent endeavour to be authentic to respondents' self-reports and at the same time attempt to reduce bias and maintain objectivity.

10.5 Recommendations

The recommendations arising from this research are categorized according to the following themes: acquisition of knowledge; integration and best practice policy; future research; individual and public health-wellness promotion. Based on insights gleaned from the findings of this research, the following recommendations are proposed:

- Have a working knowledge of Falun Gong;
- Integrate Falun Gong with counseling and other health practices;
- Provide Falun Gong practice in local community settings;
- Conduct future Falun Gong health-wellness research; and
- Develop a counseling or self-help resource.

10.5.1 Have a working knowledge of Falun Gong

The first recommendation advises counselors and other health professionals to have a working knowledge and understanding of Falun Gong to achieve effective therapeutic interactions with individuals from diverse backgrounds who may be practicing Falun Gong or similar Eastern meditative movement practices. This will help to demystify Falun Gong and minimize misconceptions about individuals who practice it. Gale and Gorman-Yao (2003) emphasized trans-cultural nursing and health care practices, and discussed the cultural implications and health-wellness potential of Falun Gong in trans-cultural nursing practice, with the need for "culturally appropriate and sensitive nursing care to all clients" (p. 124). A similar approach needs to be adopted in the counseling context as this research has shown, to enable person-centered responses, culturally and spiritually appropriate health care, and therapy for Falun Gong clients through having knowledge and sensitivity to their practice.

Barriers such as discomfort, confusion, and lack of confidence and knowledge have hindered health professionals' interactions with clients in terms of their spiritual beliefs and practices (Haynes et al., 2007; Hilbers et al., 2007). Findings from this research provide further support for the importance and consequences of culturally and spiritually sensitive health counseling services. Health professionals will not only benefit from their shared and respectful understanding of Falun Gong but also the increased awareness to attend to Falun Gong clients' general health state, if they see them.

Findings of this research have indicated that Falun Gong practitioners tend to seek professional health care services less regularly than non–Falun Gong individuals. In this context, equipped with the knowledge of Falun Gong and its healing benefits, health professionals will broaden their repertoire of strategies and services to support their non–Falun Gong clients. These professionals may consider integrating Falun Gong meditation or exercises into their counseling or support sessions, or consider inviting a Falun Gong practitioner volunteer to run a Falun Gong workshop for their clients. Based on the researcher's own professional counseling experience, this was how Falun Gong was successfully integrated and introduced to many clients at the two medical centers where the researcher was working.

10.5.2 Integrate Falun Gong with counseling and other health practices

The second recommendation offers suggestions for counselors and other health professionals regarding integrating Falun Gong into the context of their work. Integration can be achieved in several ways: 1) as an alternative self-help mind-body intervention strategy; 2) an adjunct to counseling and therapy; and 3) having knowledge and understanding of Falun Gong, and applying this in therapeutic interactions with Falun Gong and non–Falun Gong clients. Embodying the Falun Gong principles of truthfulness, compassion, and forbearance (H. Li, 2001b) with Rogers' person-centered counseling principles of accurate empathy, congruence and unconditional positive regard (Elliott & Freire, 2007; Mearns & Thorne, 2007; C. R. Rogers, 1951, 1957) in therapeutic interactions can be an effective means of working with Falun Gong and non–Falun Gong clients. These principles facilitate mutuality and respect that will, in turn, promote therapeutic interactions and relationships.

Likewise, health-wellness enhancing traits, such as optimism, positive self-perception and positive righteous thoughts that characterized the Falun Gong respondents in this research can be utilized in working with all clients. Other concepts such as positive psychology, motivational interviews, multicultural, and transpersonal approaches to counseling can also be integrated into therapeutic interactions with Falun Gong and non–Falun Gong clients, and be of benefit to, and enhance their health and wellness.

Because Falun Gong focuses on cultivating the main consciousness, therapeutic techniques, such cognitive behavior therapy, choice theory and reality therapy, journal work, self-observation diary, and others that involve cognition, rationalization of behavior, thought, and feeling patterns can be effectively integrated into the therapeutic interactions for supporting Falun Gong clients. This enables the counselor (and other health professionals) to gain an insight into issues, which Falun Gong clients regard as attachments and hence undesirable behavioral patterns to be eliminated during the Falun Gong cultivation process or through therapeutic interactions.

10.5.3 Provide Falun Gong practice in local community settings

Meditation, tai chi and yoga classes are often provided in local community settings. Hence this third recommendation pertains to the health-wellness potential of Falun Gong, its health cost savings, and the provision of Falun Gong meditation sessions in local community settings where desired or needed. "Sometimes the best things in life are free" (Oz, 2003, p. 2). Practicing Falun Gong is free of charge. Unlike other meditative practices, individuals who wish to learn and practice Falun Gong are not required to pay fees. Volunteer assistants (or Falun Gong exercise instructors) are not allowed to charge a fee. This was stipulated as one of the requirements of spreading the practice:

> The first one is that you cannot collect a fee. ... If you collect a fee ... you will no longer be a practitioner of our Falun Dafa. What you spread will not be our Falun Dafa. When you spread it, you should not pursue fame and personal gain, but should serve others voluntarily. All practitioners are doing it this way nationwide, and assistants from different regions have also set this example themselves. If you want to learn our practice, you may come as long as you want to learn it. We can be responsible to you and will not charge you a penny (H. Li, 2001b, p. 140).

Falun Gong can thus be offered as an effective, free of charge, beneficial, mind-body health-wellness maintenance activity for people of all ages from all walks of life. It can have great health/medical cost-saving benefits for the individual and the ageing society. Although health-wellness promotion is not the ultimate goal of the practice, Falun Gong classes can be encouraged in local community centers, like other meditative movement practices such as yoga, tai chi, and meditation, for those referred by health professionals or others seeking a self-help practice for overall mind-body spiritual health-wellness improvement. Findings of this research could help support applications for community grants to cover basic costs such as rental space for Falun Gong classes to cater to the needs of local residents.

10.5.4 Conduct future health-wellness Falun Gong research

This Australian-based research is the first of its kind and hence sets a benchmark for future Falun Gong health-wellness studies. Findings from this research indicate a positive link between Falun Gong and the health-wellness of Falun Gong respondents. However, it was not the aim and scope of this research to measure spirituality or spiritual health-wellness or to investigate a causal link between Falun Gong/spirituality and health. Like other studies (Koenig & Cohen, 2002; Rippentrop et al., 2005) examining the link between spirituality/religion and health, only co-relational data were obtainable from this cross-sectional Internet-based survey and hence no causal relationship could be established.

Future health-wellness Falun Gong studies can have a spirituality health-wellness focus and investigate any causal link between Falun Gong, spirituality and health-wellness. In order to determine causality, it is necessary to conduct randomized controlled trials, in particular, to determine the basis for the kinds of health/wellness differences found in this research and to exclude all other possible variables.

This research has also established a foundation for further and more in-depth, qualitative studies. It is recommended that future studies consider focusing on longitudinal studies, including considerations for age and gender differences, on phenomenology to explore lived experiences of Falun Gong practitioners and grounded theory research to explore the multi-dimensions of the health-wellness effects of Falun Gong. Further research should be conducted to assess the way the proposed six-step process could be integrated into the counseling practice and adopted as a self-help strategy.

10.5.5 Develop a counseling or self-help resource

This last recommendation proposes using a rational step-by-step process to help Falun Gong practitioners in the counseling context and/or in other therapeutic interactions. The six-step process is devised for all readers, counselors and other health professionals, to assist Falun Gong individuals undergoing the process of identifying and recognizing their issues, regarded as attachments and hence undesirable thoughts, emotions or behavioral patterns to be eliminated during cultivation practice. This process arises from basic and person-centered counseling skills (Egan, 1990; Howatt, 2000; Merry, 2002), the Crisis Intervention Model (James & Gilliland, 2008) and a working knowledge of the core principles of Falun Gong teachings (H. Li, 2001a, 2001b).

The following six-step process can be a self-help tool to be used by Falun Gong practitioners themselves or as a possible intervention strategy during therapeutic interactions.

The six steps comprise:
- Define the problem or difficulty;
- Externalize feelings and thoughts;
- Identify presenting issues (or attachments);
- Cultivate wellness: Assess and support;
- Examine strategies, make plans; and
- Commit to facilitate change.

This six-step process is a rational and systematic approach to help Falun Gong practitioners examine themselves and gain insight into their problems. It provides a logical sequence for identifying and overcoming issues or tribulations in the daily life of Falun Gong practitioners. However, it is not a replacement or an alternative technique to the teachings and practice of Falun Gong for current and future Falun Gong practitioners. Falun Gong practitioners should follow the teachings of Falun Gong as the guide for their cultivation practice. The six steps merely provide a step-by-step means of helping individuals understand the process involved in identifying and removing attachments.

Since looking within, identifying and letting go of attachments, and improving *xinxing* (heart-mind nature and moral character) are essential aspects of Falun Gong cultivation, this step-by-step process may be helpful for some individuals. Table 10.1 outlines the six-step process.

10.5.6 Concluding summary

This pioneering research has provided a demographic profile of Falun Gong respondents and found they are not unlike non–Falun Gong respondents. Falun Gong respondents are married with families, tertiary education qualifications, and occupations in society, like other normal law-abiding citizens, with the exception of their spiritual beliefs and practice that offer them health-wellness benefits. Just as we all have different beliefs that make each one of us unique, Falun Gong respondents are no different from non–Falun Gong respondents and other individuals. The research findings affirm that Falun Gong respondents are just like non–Falun Gong individuals and help clarify misconceptions that Falun Gong respondents might be demographically different compared to non–Falun Gong respondents. Nevertheless, findings indicate that Falun Gong respondents have better health-wellness status and are more likely to report excellent health, with no or little use of medication, and less medical and health expenses, compared to non–Falun Gong respondents. They also have more optimistic perceptions of their health than non–Falun Gong respondents. These are positive attributes that non–Falun Gong individuals can aspire to, with lessons to be learned from having a strong spiritual belief and faith in Falun Gong that offers health-wellness benefits and spiritual improvement. Findings from this research have highlighted a positive link between Falun Gong and health-wellness, although no causal relationship can be established.

With increasing health costs and stressful lifestyles, Falun Gong offers a free-of-charge mind-body health-wellness maintenance activity with great potential for all, including our ageing society. The relevance of Falun Gong to counseling psychology should not be underestimated, as counselors and other health professionals often work in diverse and multicultural settings to provide quality service and care to individuals who may practice Falun Gong or other similar meditative movement practices. Greater insight and understanding will benefit the client and the health professional alike.

Table 10.1 Six-step process for identifying and eliminating issues

---

Step One: Define the problem

Tell your story. Describe problems, scenario, or what troubles the mind and heart.

Step Two: Externalize feelings and thoughts

Express or write down positive and negative words, phrases, and sentences that best describe how you feel and think. E.g. "I feel sick in my tummy," "I feel fearful, upset, angry, worried, etc."

Step Three: Identify presenting issues (or attachments)

Identify and highlight main issues from written statements in Step Two. Be honest. Look within; examine your thoughts and behavior.

Step Four: Cultivate wellness/Support change

Facilitate change. Cultivate heart and mind. Replace negative self-talk with positive thoughts. Take tribulations as opportunity for self-improvement. Reassure, seek support and help if necessary.

Step Five: Examine strategies and make plans

Brainstorm strategies for action. Make short and medium-term action plans. Be mindful of every single thought and negate all negativity. (For practitioners, apply Falun Gong principles—righteous thoughts meditation, Fa study, and exercises—without pursuit.)

Step Six: Achieve commitment to facilitate change

Commit to a definite action plan. Review, summarize, and set goals. Make it happen. Ask what you need to do to achieve your goal. How and when you will know if your plan has been successfully implemented.

(Helpful questions to ask: "Now that you've gone through these steps, what is your goal? What specific action(s) will you take to ensure that you commit to the plan? How will you handle this issue if it reoccurs?")

Note: For Falun Gong practitioners, follow the teachings of Falun Gong. The six-steps merely explain the process one goes through to identify and eliminate issues.

(Egan, 1990; Howatt, 2000; James & Gilliland, 2008; Lau, 2010a; Merry, 2002)

Falun Gong, with its health-wellness effects as a bio-psychosocial-spiritual cultivation practice, its role as a counseling adjunct, relevance in therapeutic interactions, trans-cultural and multicultural counseling, and as an overall mind-body-spiritual self-improvement practice, is beneficial for both the present and future society. This research sets the scene for future health-wellness Falun Gong studies and endeavors to inspire researchers to undertake further Falun Gong studies.

It is hoped that this dissertation has enabled readers to think with a new frame of mind about Falun Gong and those who practice it. This dissertation concludes with the words from Lord Byron in *The Melody of the Heart*:

> *Words are things, and a small drop of ink falling like dew upon a thought produces that which makes thousands, perhaps millions, think (cited in Author Unknown, 1911, p. 113).*

Acknowledgements

In conducting this research, besides the many rewarding experiences, there have been interferences and unimaginable challenges. My initial supervisor Dr. John H. Court, also the Doctor of Counseling Program Director, described the entire journey as "such an unusual study fraught with so many obstacles along the way."

One of the greatest challenges right from the onset in 2003 was finding a supervisor. In 2005, due to the difficulty of finding one, I relinquished my plan to do this research for another topic with two other doctoral students. This was aborted within six months. Eventually, in 2006, John agreed to take on the principal supervisor role. Dr. Heather Mattner (at the time employed by the University of South Australia), who holds a keen interest in yoga and meditation, agreed to be the associate supervisor. In February 2008, when John retired, Dr. Paul Whetham, from the School of Psychology, was assigned to take over, but he left the university within a few months. Dr. Heather Mattner then took on the principal supervisor role until December 2008 when she too left for a position in another university, where she did her best to maintain supervisory contact via email communications. I had completed writing the dissertation chapters in February 2009. However, it took another ten months, going back and forth via email communications with Heather, who was initially inundated with numerous problems with her university computer, Internet and email services, and constantly losing emails or the attachments I sent her. My supervision experience in 2009 was at times like being alone in a boat on the high seas without a rudder. Eventually, in September 2009, I took an interstate trip to Southern Cross University in Tweed Heads, New South Wales, to see Heather for a worthwhile face-to-face supervision session. After that, it was another tedious rewriting process before the dissertation was ready for submission.

I encountered and endured many challenges that included repeated episodes of intimidations and an attempted assault in January 2006. This incident happened just after I resumed this research and required me to apply for a six-month leave from my studies. The various unexplained incidents stopped after we contacted the Australian Security Intelligence Organisation (ASIO) officer.

I wish to express my gratitude and appreciation to the special and dedicated individuals who have enriched my research journey in diverse ways and take this opportunity to thank them:

Associate Professor Heather Mattner, at the Southern Cross University, New South Wales, for spurring me on to do my best and providing me with unlimited support, insight, enthusiasm, and constructive feedback. She was like a ray of sunshine throughout my dissertation journey and left an indelible mark on this dissertation with her dedication to her supervisory role, despite having left the university and confronted with a busy schedule in her new role. I extend my appreciation for her guidance, feedback, sense of humor, wonderful smiling persona, dedication, and commitment to see me right through to the end of my doctoral dissertation journey.

Dr. John H. Court, for guiding me through the initial conceptualization of this research, the ethics protocol application, design of the questionnaires, implementation and data collection phase, and the initial dissertation writing process.

Associate Professor Kurt Lushington, Associate Head of the School of Psychology, for his suggestion during the research design's developmental stage in the choice of having non–Falun Gong friends and their family members as the comparison group, and for assisting with the submission of this dissertation.

Members of the university staff, including the Dean and Acting Deputy Vice-Chancellor and Associate Professor Margaret Peters, Dr. Jonathan Crichton, Dr. Nadine Pelling, Dr. Paul Whetham, Dr. Peter Winwood, and fellow members of the Doctor of Counselling program, particularly Anasuya, Rob, and Siti.

Members of the Falun Dafa associations, John Andress, John Deller, Peter Jauhal, and Dr Michael Pearson-Smith; pilot study team members Dr. J. Y. Luo, Dr. Y. Luo, Peter and Wendy Tiong, and Michael Tsang; Adelaide Falun Dafa practitioners, especially Sheaumay Chang, Dr. J. J. Lu, Barbara and Brian Thompson; also Trisha Anderson, Paul Robert Burton, Joe Ralli, Matthew Robertson, Leigh Smith, April

Sun, Gerard Traub, and all respondents who participated in the research. I remain grateful and indebted to Peter Tiong and Michael Tsang for their constant and unwavering support.

My adolescent and adult clients, who welcomed and benefited from the integration of Falun Gong with counseling and crisis intervention (individual and group), and participants of the 2002 Total Health and Wellness Falun Gong project (funded by the City of Unley, South Australia), for inspiring me to undertake this research.

My brothers and especially my sister Cathy for her continual support; my late father, who believed that I would make it; and my beloved mother, who patiently waited for the day that I would complete this dissertation journey. Others included Manager Steve Denholm, and work colleagues at Transitional Accommodation, Families SA, Department for Families and Communities, for their support and being flexible with my work hours. And my dear friends, especially Valma Gay, Peggy Lim, Sonia Tay, Florence Teo, and Veronica Ting, who patiently listened to my dissertation writing woes and cheered me on to the finishing line.

As a student and practitioner of Falun Gong, I am grateful for the insights gleaned from studying the teachings of Falun Gong that have continuously provided me with the physical, emotional, and spiritual resources to enable me to complete this journey. Readers, please keep in mind that this research is merely scratching the surface and that greater knowledge of and insight into Falun Gong can only be gained through reading the teachings of Falun Gong. I remain infinitely grateful for the miracles along the way, specifically the amazing recovery of my eyesight that enabled me to spend long hours each day in front of my 13-inch laptop. I had a congenital eye condition in both eyes and never had dual eye vision for most of my life. After four eye surgeries, I gradually lost vision in one eye to about 10%. During my busiest dissertation writing time, I regained good dual eye vision. Now I enjoy stable dual eye vision without any eyestrain.

I would like to conclude with the words from one of my favorite Robert Frost's poem, *The Road Not Taken*:

> *Two roads diverged in a wood, and I—I took the one less travelled by. And that has made all the difference. (Frost, 1969, p. 105)*

Appendix 1: Letter to Participants

18 June 2007

Dear participant

My name is Margaret Lau and I am a doctoral candidate at the University of South Australia. I am seeking volunteers for a research study to investigate the effect of Falun Gong (also known as Falun Dafa) on individuals who practise this meditation form. This study is undertaken as part of my Professional Doctorate in Counselling.

The purpose of this survey is to gain a snapshot of the demographics of Falun Gong practitioners around the world, to study the impact of the practice on individuals' health and wellbeing as perceived and reported by practitioners, and how that compares with people who do not practise Falun Gong or similar practices and other forms of meditation.

I would like to invite Falun Gong practitioners to contribute to this online survey. To participate fully in this survey, you also need to invite a friend, or a family member, to complete the survey. This person must not be practising Falun Gong or other meditation on a daily or regular basis during the past 6 months. For participation criteria, please refer to the Research Information Sheet (RIS).

Participation is entirely voluntary. You and your invited friend, or family member, are under no obligation to participate in the survey. All responses are confidential and anonymous. No one can be identified or identifiable in this survey. The researcher will take every care to remove responses from any identifying material as early as possible. All responses will be kept confidential by the researcher and not be identified in the reporting of the research. Please do not complete the online survey if participating poses a security risk for you and your family.

The University's Human Research Ethics Committee (HREC) has reviewed and approved this study. If you have any ethical concerns about the project or questions about your rights as a participant, please contact the Executive Officer of this Committee, Tel: +61 8 8302 3118; Email: vicki.allen@unisa.edu.au.

The Australian and the European Falun Dafa Associations have approved for the research information and survey web links to be posted on their web sites.

I hope you will take this opportunity to participate and to give a self-report of the impact of Falun Gong in your life. Should you require further information, please contact me, or my supervisor.

Yours sincerely,

Project Researcher
Margaret Lau
Doctor of Counselling Candidate
School of Psychology, Playford Building
University of South Australia
North Terrace, Adelaide
SA 5000 AUSTRALIA
margaret.lau@postgrads.unisa.edu.au

Principal Supervisor
Dr John Court
School of Psychology, Playford Building
University of South Australia
North Terrace, Adelaide
SA 5000 AUSTRALIA
Tel: 61 8 8302 1016   Fax: 61 8 8302 2959
john.court@unisa.edu.au

Appendix 2: Research Information Sheet (RIS)

Research Information Sheet (RIS)

Survey of the Effect of Falun Gong on Health and Wellness

Purpose of the Study

This research investigates the effects of Falun Gong on health and the maintenance of existing wellness from the self-reports of individuals who practise Falun Gong as contrasted with those who do not practise Falun Gong or similar practices and other forms of meditation.

The aim is to gain a snapshot of the demographics of Falun Gong practitioners, to study the impact of the practice on individuals' health and wellbeing as perceived by practitioners, and how that compares with people who do not practise Falun Gong or other forms of meditation.

Falun Gong is better known as Falun Dafa. For consistency, Falun Gong is used in all research materials.

Value

There is a growing awareness in the West of self-help meditative practices from Eastern cultures. These self-improvement therapies like Yoga, Tai Chi and Qigong practices share common characteristics and are traditionally valued for better health and wellness outcomes.

While there is substantial literature on Yoga, Tai Chi, and other forms of qigong, little research has been done on the efficacy of Falun Gong. This is despite the fact that the practice has attracted tens of millions of people from over 80 countries. Many gain better health, inner peace and joy from the practice. A survey conducted in Beijing (1998), with over 12,000 respondents indicated that Falun Gong has a significant effect in promoting physical and mental health and enhancing wellness.

This Australian-based research will be the first worldwide demographic survey involving a comparative sample. The value of the proposed study is that it will explore the potential for Falun Gong to improve the health and wellbeing of practitioners. It will augment existing limited research on Falun Gong and offers insight into its role as a body-mind intervention, self-improvement therapy and spiritual practice.

By participating, you will be contributing to the study on how Falun Gong affects health and wellness, and the degree to which this meditation practice makes a pivotal difference in your life. Findings of the survey will assist in validating the role of Falun Gong in maintaining health and wellness. It will also provide insights into the wider implications of the significance of Falun Gong practice in the promotion of body-mind health and wellness and as a form of group intervention strategy for better health and wellness outcomes for the public, contemporary and future society.

Design and Methodology

The study addresses the following research question:

Effects of Falun Gong: Whether the practice affects the health and wellbeing of practitioners.

To investigate this question, the study will use a quantitative method with anonymous questionnaires administered via Internet. The study consists of the following three phases:

1. Participant identification: This online survey is open to Falun Gong practitioners around the world. There are two groups of participants; (1) individuals who identify themselves as Falun Gong practitioners and (2) individuals who do not practise Falun Gong, or other type of meditation practice in the past 6 months and who are invited by practitioners to do the survey.

2. Data collection: A time frame of 5+ weeks will be set for data collection. There are two questionnaires. Health & Wellness Survey One is for Falun Gong practitioners; Health & Wellness Survey Two is for non-practitioners. Letter to participants, Research Information Sheet (RIS) and web links for the two surveys will be posted on the Australian and European Falun Dafa websites. There is no restriction placed on the number of participants completing survey.

3. Data analysis: Data collected will be analysed using the Statistical Package for Social Sciences (SPSS). A summary of the findings will be published on Falun Dafa websites and a subsequent date will be announced for the completion of the final research report.

Research Information Sheet (RIS)

Participation Criteria

1. **HW Survey One:** You must be a Falun Gong practitioner for more than 6 months, engaging in regular and consistent daily/weekly practice of the exercises and study of Falun Gong teachings.

2. **HW Survey Two:** One friend or family member invited by Falun Gong practitioners. He/She must NOT be practising Falun Gong, meditation, or similar practices, e.g. tai chi, qigong, yoga on a regular (daily/weekly) basis during the past 6 months. Ideally, this person is from your age range.

    18 – 29 years; 30 – 39 years; 40 – 49 years; 50 – 59 years; 60 – 69 years; Above 70 years

3. Failure to invite a non-Falun Gong practitioner to do the HW2 Survey will not disqualify you from participation. However, please do your best to meet this criterion.

4. **Participation is voluntary.** No one is under any obligation to do the survey. The researcher will not be approaching Falun Gong practitioners in China. Please do not complete the online survey if Falun Gong is banned in your country, or if participating poses a security risk for you and your family.

Research Process & Instructions

1. **All participants should try to complete the survey online.** The process should take about 20 minutes. Please give yourself enough time to complete the entire survey.

2. **There are two surveys.** Health & Wellness Survey 1 for Falun Gong practitioners (HW1); Health & Wellness Survey 2 for Non-Falun Gong Practitioners (HW2), i.e. individuals – friends and family members who do not practise Falun Gong, or other similar practices. The web links for both surveys will be placed on the Australian and European Falun Dafa websites.

3. **The online survey is in English.** Translated Chinese versions of the surveys are available for printing and to help respondents to complete the online survey. You may seek help from practitioners/friends to complete the survey.

4. The web links for the surveys will be posted by 28 June 2007. To do the surveys, please visit www.falunau.org or www.clearharmony.com

5. Under **exceptional circumstances**, if you are unable to complete the online survey, you can complete and submit a paper version to Margaret Lau, c/o Dr John Court and post it to the address given below. The researcher will then use an independent third party to electronically input data.

Participants' responses will be kept confidential and unidentified in the research report. Researchers, however, cannot guarantee the confidentiality or anonymity of material transferred by email or Internet. Every care will be taken to separate responses from any identifying material as early as possible.

Hard copies of summarized results will be stored in lockable filing cabinets in the School of Psychology. All data and summarised results will also be stored on computers with CD backups in a lockable cabinet by the researcher. The recorded data will be securely stored for a minimum of 7 years in accordance with the Australian Freedom of Information legislation.

The University's Human Research Ethics Committee (HREC) has reviewed this study. If you have any ethical concerns about the project or questions about your rights as a participant, please contact the Executive Officer of this Committee, Tel: +61 8 8302 3118; Email: vicki.allen@unisa.edu.au.

Thank you for your contribution and help with the survey.

Project Researcher
Margaret Lau
Doctor of Counselling Candidate
School of Psychology, Playford Building
University of South Australia
North Terrace
Adelaide SA 5000 AUSTRALIA
margaret.lau@postgrads.unisa.edu.au

Principal Supervisor
Dr John Court
School of Psychology, Playford Building
University of South Australia
North Terrace
Adelaide SA 5000 AUSTRALIA
Tel: 61 8 8302 1016   Fax: 61 8 8302 2959
john.court@unisa.edu.au

Appendix 3: Health and Wellness Survey One (HW1)

Health & Wellness Survey One for Falun Gong Practitioners (HW1)

Dear participant,
This is the Health & Wellness Survey (HW1) for Falun Gong practitioners. Your participation will help in the study of the effect of Falun Gong practice on health and wellness as compared with people who don't practise Falun Gong or other forms of meditation.
The online survey takes 20 minutes. Please read all instructions carefully and set aside enough time to complete the survey.
Participation is voluntary. You are under no obligation to participate. The researcher will not be approaching Falun Gong practitioners in China. Please do not complete this survey if Falun Gong is banned in your country, or if participating poses a security risk for you and your family.
All responses are confidential, anonymous, and no one will be identified. (However, the researcher cannot guarantee the confidentiality or anonymity of material transferred by email or Internet.)
Please complete each question before going to the next question.

SECTION 1 - ABOUT YOU:

The questions in the first section provide information on the global demographic characteristics of respondents.
To respond, please place a check ☒ in the box or click the button next to the most appropriate option.

1. Are you ☐ Male or ☐ Female?

2. Which age group do you belong to?
   ☐ Under 20 years
   ☐ 20 – 29 years
   ☐ 30 – 39 years
   ☐ 40 – 49 years
   ☐ 50 – 59 years
   ☐ 60 – 69 years
   ☐ 70 years and above

3. What is your relationship status?
   ☐ Now married
   ☐ De facto relationship (Cohabitation)
   ☐ Never married
   ☐ Divorced/Separated
   ☐ Widowed

4. How do you identify your ethnicity? Please specify. (E.g. Australian Aboriginal, African, Arabic, Chinese, Hispanic or Mediterranean, Indian, Japanese, Northern European and Slav, Sri Lankan, South Sea Islander, etc.)

   ……………………...................…………

5. What is your country of birth? (E.g. Australia, Canada, China, France, India, Italy, Malaysia, Sweden, Taiwan, UK, USA, Vietnam, etc.)

   ……………………...................…………

6. What is your current country of residence? (E.g. Australia, Canada, China, France, India, Italy, Malaysia, Sweden, Taiwan, UK, USA, etc.)

   ……………………...................…………

7. Is English your first language? (The language you grew up with as a child)
   ☐ Yes ☐ No

8. If English is not your first language, what is your first language? (E.g. Chinese Mandarin, Chinese Dialect, French, Italian, Bahasa Malaysia, Portuguese, Russian, Spanish, Vietnamese, etc.)

   ……………………...................…………

9. What is your highest educational attainment?
   ☐ Middle/Secondary/Primary School
   ☐ High/Senior School Diploma or equivalent
   ☐ Undergraduate degree (bachelor)
   ☐ Master or postgraduate degree
   ☐ PhD or Doctoral degree

10. What is your current occupation? (E.g. chef, counsellor, lawyer, medical doctor, plumber, secretary, police or secret agent, college or university student, retired, etc.)

    ……………………...................…………

11. What is your gross annual household income? [in your local currency, for e.g. Yen180,000, US$80,000, 100,000 rupees, £38,000]

    ……………………...................…………

Health & Wellness Survey One for Falun Gong Practitioners (HW1)

SECTION 2 – YOUR MEDICAL HISTORY AND HEALTH STATUS

12. How many times have you consulted a medical doctor during the past 6 months?
    - ☐ None
    - ☐ 1 - 3 times
    - ☐ 4 - 6 times
    - ☐ 7 - 9 times
    - ☐ Over 10 times

13. If you have consulted a medical doctor, briefly state main reason(s). (E.g. bone fracture, colds.)
    ....
    ....

14. Are you currently taking any of the following? (Check ☒ all that apply)
    - ☐ None
    - ☐ Prescription drugs (medical)
    - ☐ Over counter drugs, e.g. Panadol, Aspirin
    - ☐ Chinese herbal remedies
    - ☐ Western herbal remedies
    - ☐ Homeopathic remedies
    - ☐ Multi-vitamins and health supplements

15. How much have you spent on all medical and health expenses (including prescriptions, herbal remedies, supplements) in the past six months? Write *None* or state total amount [in your local currency, e.g. US$500, 10,000 rupees, etc.]
    ....

16. Do you smoke tobacco cigarettes?
    - ☐ No
    - ☐ Yes

17. If yes, how many cigarettes per day? (E.g. 20 cigarettes per day.) ....

18. Do you plan to stop smoking?
    - ☐ No
    - ☐ Yes
    - ☐ Not Applicable

19. Do you consume alcohol? ☐ No   ☐ Yes

20. If yes, how much alcohol per day? (E.g. 50mls spirits, 200mls wine, 500mls beer.)
    ....

21. Do you plan to stop consuming alcohol?
    - ☐ No
    - ☐ Yes
    - ☐ Not Applicable

22. Do you use recreational drugs (e.g. heroin, ice, marijuana, ecstasy, etc.)?
    - ☐ No
    - ☐ Yes

23. If yes, what recreational drug(s) do you use?
    ....

24. Do you plan to stop using recreational drugs?
    - ☐ No
    - ☐ Yes
    - ☐ Not Applicable

SECTION 3: MEDITATION PRACTICE

25. What is Falun Gong? Check ☒ the most appropriate option.
    - ☐ It is a form of religion with its origin from Buddhist teachings
    - ☐ Also known as Falun Dafa, it is an advanced cultivation practice based on truthfulness, compassion and forbearance
    - ☐ It is a type of Qigong practice
    - ☐ It is a sect based on Taoist and Buddhist teachings
    - ☐ Don't know

26. Which of the following is MOST important in the practice of Falun Gong?
    - ☐ Practise the exercises daily
    - ☐ Study teachings of Falun Gong
    - ☐ Maintain a positive attitude
    - ☐ Organise experience sharing conference
    - ☐ Don't know

27. How long have you practised Falun Gong?
    - ☐ 6 months-2 years
    - ☐ 2-4 years
    - ☐ 4-6 years
    - ☐ 6-8 years
    - ☐ 8 –10 years
    - ☐ Over 10 years

28. How often do you practise the exercises?
    - ☐ Once a week
    - ☐ 2-3 times a week
    - ☐ 4-5 times a week
    - ☐ Daily

29. Please state time spent on the practice for each session.
    - ☐ 30 minutes
    - ☐ 1 hour
    - ☐ 1 hour 30 minutes
    - ☐ 2 hours

30. How often do you study the teachings of Falun Gong?
    - ☐ Once a week
    - ☐ 2-3 times a week
    - ☐ 4-5 times a week
    - ☐ Daily

31. Please state total time spent on the study each week.
    - ☐ None
    - ☐ 1 - 5 hours
    - ☐ 6 – 10 hours
    - ☐ 11 - 15 hours
    - ☐ 16 - 20 hours
    - ☐ Over 20 hours

32. How has your physical health changed since practising Falun Gong?
    - ☐ Significantly worse
    - ☐ Slightly worse
    - ☐ No difference
    - ☐ Slightly improved
    - ☐ Significantly improved

Health & Wellness Survey One for Falun Gong Practitioners (HW1)

33. How has your mental and emotional health changed since practising Falun Gong?
    - ☐ Significantly worse
    - ☐ Slightly worse
    - ☐ No difference
    - ☐ Slightly improved
    - ☐ Significantly improved

34. How has your stress coping ability changed since practising Falun Gong?
    - ☐ Significantly worse
    - ☐ Slightly worse
    - ☐ No difference
    - ☐ Slightly improved
    - ☐ Significantly improved

35. How has your relationship with significant others changed since practising Falun Gong?
    - ☐ Significantly worse
    - ☐ Slightly worse
    - ☐ No difference
    - ☐ Slightly improved
    - ☐ Significantly improved

36. How has your attitude to life changed since practising Falun Gong?
    - ☐ Significantly worse
    - ☐ Slightly worse
    - ☐ No difference
    - ☐ Slightly improved
    - ☐ Significantly improved

37. Did you have any medical condition(s) as diagnosed by medical doctors before practising Falun Gong?   ☐ No   ☐ Yes

38. If yes, please specify, e.g. anxiety disorder, lung cancer, heart disease, chronic fatigue/pain, etc.

    ....
    ....

39. How would you rate your medical condition since practising Falun Gong?
    - ☐ Significantly worse
    - ☐ Slightly worse
    - ☐ No difference
    - ☐ Slightly improved
    - ☐ Significantly improved
    - ☐ Not Applicable

Please check ☒ Not Applicable if Q 40 & 41 don't apply to you.

40. If you smoked tobacco cigarettes before you started Falun Gong practice, did you stop the smoking habit after starting practice?

☐ No   ☐ Yes   ☐ Not Applicable

41. If you drank alcohol before you started Falun Gong practice, did you stop your alcohol consumption since starting practice?
    ☐ No   ☐ Yes   ☐ Not Applicable

42. What first attracted you to Falun Gong practice? Select THREE that most apply.
    - ☐ Search for meaning in life
    - ☐ Family/friends practise Falun Gong
    - ☐ Falun Gong exercises
    - ☐ Teachings of Falun Gong
    - ☐ Spiritual enlightenment offered by Falun Gong
    - ☐ Physical and Mental Health Benefits
    - ☐ A predestined relationship (e.g. I just knew this is for me.)
    - ☐ Other

43. Please specify or explain what you mean by "Other" in Question 42.

    ....
    ....

44. How do you think Falun Gong practice has led to better health and wellness in your life? Check ☒ THREE that most apply.
    - ☐ Falun Gong exercise routine
    - ☐ Regular study of Falun Gong teachings
    - ☐ Falun Gong community
    - ☐ Improved stress coping ability
    - ☐ Positive change of attitude towards life since practising Falun Gong
    - ☐ Improving xinxing or moral character based on the principles of Truthfulness, Compassion and Forbearance.
    - ☐ Falun Gong experience sharing conferences
    - ☐ Other

45. Please specify or explain what you mean by "Other" in Question 44.

    ....
    ....

SECTION 4:   THE SF36 HEALTH SURVEY

Please turn the page and complete Section 4.

Health & Wellness Survey One for Falun Gong Practitioners (HW1)

SECTION 4: SF36 HEALTH SURVEY

INSTRUCTIONS: This set of questions asks for your views about your health. This information will help keep track of how you feel and how well you are able to do your usual activities. Answer every question by marking the answer as indicated. If you are unsure about how to answer a question please give the best answer you can.

46. In general, would you say your health is: (Please check ☒ one box.)

Excellent	☐
Very Good	☐
Good	☐
Fair	☐
Poor	☐

47. Compared to one year ago, how would you rate your health in general now? (Please check ☒ one box.)

Much better than one year ago	☐
Somewhat better than last year	☐
About the same as one year ago	☐
Somewhat worse now than one year ago	☐
Much worse than one year ago	☐

The following questions are about activities you might do during a typical day. Does your health now limit you in these activities? If so, how much. **(Please circle one number on each line.)**

Activities	Yes, Limited A Lot	Yes, Limited A Little	Not Limited At All
48. a. **Vigorous activities**, such as running, lifting heavy objects, participating in strenuous sports	1	2	3
49. b. **Moderate activities**, such as moving a table, pushing a vacuum cleaner, bowling, or playing golf	1	2	3
50. c. Lifting or carrying groceries	1	2	3
51. d. Climbing **several** flights of stairs	1	2	3
52. e. Climbing **one** flight of stairs	1	2	3
53. f. Bending, kneeling, or stooping	1	2	3
54. g. Walking **more than a mile**	1	2	3
55. h. Walking **several** blocks	1	2	3
56. i. Walking **one block**	1	2	3
57. j. Bathing or dressing yourself	1	2	3

During the past 4 weeks, have you had any of the following problems with your work or other regular daily activities as a result of your physical health? **(Please circle one number on each line.)**

	Yes	No
58. a. Cut down on the **amount of time** you spent on work or other activities	1	2
59. b. Accomplished less than you would like	1	2
60. c. Were **limited** in the **kind** of work or other activities	1	2
61. d. Had **difficulty** performing the work or other activities	1	2

During the past 4 weeks, have you had any of the following problems with your work or other regular daily activities as a result of any emotional problems (e.g. feeling depressed or anxious)?
(Please circle one number on each line.)

	Yes	No
62. a. Cut down on the **amount of time** you spent on work or other activities	1	2
63. b. Accomplished less than you would like	1	2
64. c. Didn't do work or other activities **as carefully** as usual	1	2

Health & Wellness Survey One for Falun Gong Practitioners (HW1)

65. During the <u>past 4 weeks</u>, to what extent has your physical health or emotional problems interfered with your normal social activities with family, friends, neighbours, or groups? (Please check ☒ **one** box.)

Not at all ☐
Slightly ☐
Moderately ☐
Quite a bit ☐
Extremely ☐

66. How much physical pain have you had during the past 4 weeks? (Please check ☒ **one** box.)

None ☐   Mild ☐   Moderate ☐
Severe ☐   Very Severe ☐

67. During the <u>past 4 weeks</u>, how much did pain interfere with your normal work (including both work outside the home and housework? (Please check ☒ **one** box.)

Not at all ☐
Slightly ☐
Moderately ☐
Quite a bit ☐
Extremely ☐

These questions are about how your feel and how things have been with you <u>during the past 4 weeks</u>. Please give the one answer that is closest to the way you have been feeling for each item.

(Please circle one number on each line.)	All of the Time	Most of the Time	A Good Bit of the Time	Some of the Time	A Little of the Time	None of the Time
68. a. Did you feel full of life?	1	2	3	4	5	6
69. b. Have you been a very nervous person?	1	2	3	4	5	6
70. c. Have you felt so down in the dumps that nothing could cheer you up?	1	2	3	4	5	6
71. d. Have you felt calm and peaceful?	1	2	3	4	5	6
72. e. Did you have a lot of energy?	1	2	3	4	5	6
73. f. Have you felt downhearted and blue?	1	2	3	4	5	6
74. g. Did you feel worn out?	1	2	3	4	5	6
75. h. Have you been a happy person?	1	2	3	4	5	6
76. i. Did you feel tired?	1	2	3	4	5	6

77. During the <u>past 4 weeks</u>, how much of the time has your physical health or emotional problems interfered with your social activities (like visiting friends, relatives, etc.) (Please check ☒ **one** box.)

All of the time ☐
Most of the time ☐
Some of the time ☐
A little of the time ☐
None of the time ☐

How TRUE or FALSE is <u>each</u> of the following statements for you?

(Please circle one number on each line.)	Definitely True	Mostly True	Don't Know	Mostly False	Definitely False
78. a. I seem to get sick a little easier than other people	1	2	3	4	5
79. b. I am as healthy as anybody I know	1	2	3	4	5
80. c. I expect my health to get worse	1	2	3	4	5
81. d. My health is excellent	1	2	3	4	5

Thank you for completing all <u>FOUR</u> sections of the survey. Your contribution to this research study project is much appreciated. If participating in this study has caused you <u>concern or worry</u>, please speak to fellow practitioners or the coordinator in your region. Or you could contact the researcher via email: margaret.lau@postgrads.unisa.edu.au. Margaret Lau, Doctor of Counselling Candidate, School of Psychology, University of South Australia, Adelaide.

228

Appendix 4: Health and Wellness Survey Two (HW2)

Health & Wellness Survey for Non-Falun Gong Practitioners (HW2)

Dear participant,
This is the Health & Wellness Survey (HW2) for respondents who do <u>NOT</u> practise Falun Gong, other meditation or similar practices such as Tai Chi, Yoga, etc. on a regular basis during the last 6 months.
This online survey will take about 15-20 minutes. Please read all instructions carefully and set aside enough time to complete the survey.
Participation is voluntary. You are under no obligation to participate in the survey. The researcher will <u>not</u> be approaching participants in China. Please do <u>not</u> complete the survey if participating poses a security risk for you and your family.
All responses are confidential and anonymous. No one will be identified or identifiable in this survey. (However, researchers cannot guarantee the security of material transferred by email or Internet.)
Please complete each question before going to the next question.

………………………....................…………

SECTION 1 - ABOUT YOU

The questions in the first section provide information on the global demographic characteristics of respondents.
To respond, please place a check ☒ in the box or click the button next to the most appropriate option.

1. Are you ☐ Male or ☐ Female?

2. Which age group do you belong to?
☐ Under 20 years
☐ 20 – 29 years
☐ 30 – 39 years
☐ 40 – 49 years
☐ 50 – 59 years
☐ 60 – 69 years
☐ 70 years and above

3. What is your relationship status?
☐ Now married
☐ De facto relationship (Cohabitation)
☐ Never married
☐ Divorced/Separated
☐ Widowed

4. How do you identify your ethnicity? Please specify. (E.g. Australian Aboriginal, African, Arabic, Chinese, Hispanic or Mediterranean, Indian, Japanese, Northern European and Slav, Sri Lankan, South Sea Islander, etc.)

………………………....................…………

5. What is your country of birth? (E.g. Australia, Canada, China, France, India, Italy, Malaysia, Sweden, Taiwan, UK, USA, Vietnam, etc.)

6. What is your current country of residence? (E.g. Australia, Canada, China, France, India, Italy, Malaysia, Sweden, Taiwan, UK, USA, etc.)

………………………....................…………

7. Is English your first language? (The language you grew up with as a child)
☐ Yes ☐ No

8. If English is <u>not</u> your first language, what is your first language? (E.g. Chinese Mandarin, Chinese Dialect, French, Italian, Bahasa Malaysia, Portuguese, Russian, Spanish, Vietnamese, etc.)

………………………....................…………

9. What is your highest educational attainment?
☐ Middle/Secondary/Primary School
☐ High/Senior School Diploma or equivalent
☐ Undergraduate degree (bachelor)
☐ Master or postgraduate degree
☐ PhD or Doctoral degree

10. What is your current occupation? (E.g. chef, counsellor, lawyer, medical doctor, plumber, secretary, police or secret agent, college or university student, retired, etc.)

………………………....................…………

11. What is your gross annual household income? [in your local currency, for e.g. Yen180,000, US$80,000, 100,000 rupees, £38,000]

………………………....................…………

Health & Wellness Survey for Non-Falun Gong Practitioners (HW2)

SECTION 2 – YOUR MEDICAL HISTORY AND HEALTH STATUS

12. How many times have you consulted a medical doctor during the past 6 months?
- [ ] None
- [ ] 1 - 3 times
- [ ] 4 - 6 times
- [ ] 7 - 9 times
- [ ] Over 10 times

13. If you have consulted a medical doctor, briefly state main reason(s). (E.g. bone fracture, colds.)
....
....

14. Are you currently taking any of the following? (Check ⊠ all that apply)
- [ ] None
- [ ] Prescription drugs (medical)
- [ ] Over counter drugs, e.g. Panadol, Aspirin
- [ ] Chinese herbal remedies
- [ ] Western herbal remedies
- [ ] Homeopathic remedies
- [ ] Multi-vitamins and health supplements

15. How much have you spent on all medical and health expenses (including prescriptions, herbal remedies, supplements) in the past six months?

....

Write *None* or state total amount [in your local currency, e.g. US$500, 10,000 rupees, etc.]

16. Do you smoke tobacco cigarettes?
- [ ] No
- [ ] Yes

17. If yes, how many cigarettes per day? (E.g. 20 cigarettes per day.) ....

18. Do you plan to stop smoking?
- [ ] No
- [ ] Yes
- [ ] Not Applicable

19. Do you consume alcohol? [ ] No [ ] Yes

20. If yes, how much alcohol per day? (E.g. 50mls spirits, 200mls wine, 500mls beer.)
....

21. Do you plan to stop consuming alcohol?
- [ ] No
- [ ] Yes
- [ ] Not Applicable

22. Do you use recreational drugs (e.g. heroin, ice, marijuana, ecstasy, etc.)?
- [ ] No
- [ ] Yes

23. If yes, what recreational drug(s) do you use?
....

24. Do you plan to stop using recreational drugs?
- [ ] No
- [ ] Yes
- [ ] Not Applicable

SECTION 3 – THE SF36 HEALTH SURVEY

INSTRUCTIONS: This set of questions asks for your views about your health. This information will help keep track of how you feel and how well you are able to do your usual activities. Answer every question by marking the answer as indicated. If you are unsure about how to answer a question please give the best answer you can.

25. In general, would you say your health is: (Please check ⊠ one box.)
- Excellent [ ]
- Very Good [ ]
- Good [ ]
- Fair [ ]
- Poor [ ]

26. Compared to one year ago, how would you rate your health in general now? (Please check ⊠ one box.)
- Much better than one year ago [ ]
- Somewhat better than last year [ ]
- About the same as one year ago [ ]
- Somewhat worse now than one year ago [ ]
- Much worse than one year ago [ ]

The following questions are about activities you might do during a typical day. Does your health now limit you in

Health & Wellness Survey for Non-Falun Gong Practitioners (HW2)

these activities? If so, how much. **(Please circle one number on each line.)**			
Activities	**Yes, Limited A Lot**	**Yes, Limited A Little**	**Not Limited At All**
27. a. **Vigorous activities**, such as running, lifting heavy objects, participating in strenuous sports	1	2	3
28. b. **Moderate activities**, such as moving a table, pushing a vacuum cleaner, bowling, or playing golf	1	2	3
29. c. Lifting or carrying groceries	1	2	3
30. d. Climbing **several** flights of stairs	1	2	3
31. e. Climbing **one** flight of stairs	1	2	3
32. f. Bending, kneeling, or stooping	1	2	3
33. g. Walking **more than a mile**	1	2	3
34. h. Walking **several** blocks	1	2	3
35. i. Walking **one block**	1	2	3
36. j. Bathing or dressing yourself	1	2	3

During the past 4 weeks, have you had any of the following problems with your work or other regular daily activities as a result of your physical health? **(Please circle one number on each line.)**	Yes	No
37. a. Cut down on the **amount of time** you spent on work or other activities	1	2
38. b. Accomplished less than you would like	1	2
39. c. Were **limited** in the **kind** of work or other activities	1	2
40. d. Had **difficulty** performing the work or other activities	1	2

During the past 4 weeks, have you had any of the following problems with your work or other regular daily activities as a result of any emotional problems (e.g. feeling depressed or anxious)? **(Please circle one number on each line.)**	Yes	No
41. a. Cut down on the **amount of time** you spent on work or other activities	1	2
42. b. Accomplished less than you would like	1	2
43. c. Didn't do work or other activities **as carefully** as usual	1	2

44. During the past 4 weeks, to what extent has your physical health or emotional problems interfered with your normal social activities with family, friends, neighbours, or groups? (Please check ☒ **one** box.)

Not at all ☐
Slightly ☐
Moderately ☐
Quite a bit ☐
Extremely ☐

45. How much physical pain have you had during the past 4 weeks? (Please check ☒ **one** box.)

None ☐   Mild ☐   Moderate ☐
Severe ☐   Very Severe ☐

46. During the past 4 weeks, how much did pain interfere with your normal work (including both work outside the home and housework? (Please check ☒ **one** box.)

Not at all ☐
Slightly ☐
Moderately ☐
Quite a bit ☐
Extremely ☐

These questions are about how your feel and how things have been with you during the past 4 weeks. Please

Health & Wellness Survey for Non-Falun Gong Practitioners (HW2)

give the one answer that is closest to the way you have been feeling for each item.

(Please circle one number on each line.)	All of the Time	Most of the Time	A Good Bit of the Time	Some of the Time	A Little of the Time	None of the Time
47. a. Did you feel full of life?	1	2	3	4	5	6
48. b. Have you been a very nervous person?	1	2	3	4	5	6
49. c. Have you felt so down in the dumps that nothing could cheer you up?	1	2	3	4	5	6
50. d. Have you felt calm and peaceful?	1	2	3	4	5	6
51. e. Did you have a lot of energy?	1	2	3	4	5	6
52. f. Have you felt downhearted and blue?	1	2	3	4	5	6
53. g. Did you feel worn out?	1	2	3	4	5	6
54. h. Have you been a happy person?	1	2	3	4	5	6
55. i. Did you feel tired?	1	2	3	4	5	6

56. During the past 4 weeks, how much of the time has your physical health or emotional problems interfered with your social activities (like visiting friends, relatives, etc.) (Please check ☒ one box.)

All of the time ☐
Most of the time ☐
Some of the time ☐
A little of the time ☐
None of the time ☐

How TRUE or FALSE is each of the following statements for you?

(Please circle one number on each line.)	Definitely True	Mostly True	Don't Know	Mostly False	Definitely False
57. a. I seem to get sick a little easier than other people	1	2	3	4	5
58. b. I am as healthy as anybody I know	1	2	3	4	5
59. c. I expect my health to get worse	1	2	3	4	5
60. d. My health is excellent	1	2	3	4	5

Thank you for completing all THREE sections of the Health & Wellness Survey for non-Falun Gong practitioners (HW2). Your contribution to this research project is much appreciated. If participating in this study has caused you concern or worry, please speak to your Falun Gong friend or family member who has invited you to participate. Alternatively, you could contact the researcher via email: margaret.lau@postgrads.unisa.edu.au.

Margaret Lau
Doctor of Counselling Candidate
School of Psychology
University of South Australia
Adelaide SA 5000 Australia
Email: margaret.lau@postgrads.unisa.edu.au

Appendix 5: ANZSCO Categories

Categories of occupations based on the Australian and New Zealand Standard Classification of Occupations (ANZSCO)

Category	Major Categories	Subcategories
1	Managers, CEOs & Senior Administrators	General, Specialist Managers, etc.
2	Business & Information Technology Professionals	Accountants, Auditors
		Advertising Marketing & Misc. Business Professionals
		IT Professionals, Finance Brokers, Dealers, Investment Advisers, & Planners
3	Education - Professionals	Teachers, University Professors
		Lecturers, Miscellaneous Educators
4	Health - Professionals	Medical/Dental: Specialist/General
		Nursing: Managers, Professors
		Educators, Researchers
		Midwives, Registered Nurses
		Misc./Allied/Natural Health Professionals
5	Science, Building, Transport & Engineering - Professionals	Engineers, Architects, Air & Marine Professionals, & Surveyors
6	Arts, Media, Social, Community Service, & Miscellaneous - Professionals	Counselors, Psychologists, Social Workers, Welfare, Community Service, Youth Workers, & Clergy, etc.
		Artists, Media: Photographers
		Journalists, Cameramen, etc.
		Writers, Musicians, Stage Directors,
		Dancers & Miscellaneous Professionals
7	Technicians & Trades Workers	Plumbers, Automotive, Construction, Foods, Animal, Horticultural trades, etc.

Category	Major Categories	Subcategories
		Electrical & Electronics, Carpentry
		Miscellaneous trades – Florists
8	Clerical, Sales, Administrative & Service workers	Personal Assistants, Secretaries, General Administrative, Inquiry, Sales & Numerical Clerks
9	Labourers – skilled and unskilled	Cleaners, Laundry, Factory Process Workers, Drivers, Freight Handlers, etc. Shelf Fillers, Farm, Forestry, Garden, & Miscellaneous Labourers
10	Retired/Home Duties	
11	Student	
12	Unemployed	

Source: (Australian Bureau of Statistics & Statistics New Zealand, 2006)

Glossary

Buddha	Sanskrit (ancient Indian language) word for a great enlightened person
cultivation	An Eastern concept for mind, body, and spiritual improvement
Dafa	Great Law, and short term for Falun Dafa
de	Virtue or merit; a precious white energy gained through enduring hardships and tribulations. This process is required for *xinxing* improvement and spiritual progress.
ding	A meditative state of tranquility in which the mind is empty, yet conscious.
Fa	Law or principles
Falun	Law Wheel
gong	Cultivation energy or a practice cultivating such energy
karma	A Sanskrit word meaning action or deed referring to bad or negative actions. In Falun Gong teachings, it is described as a black substance or energy field that is the opposite of *de.*
qi	Life force or vital energy that is present in all beings. In Falun Gong teachings, it is considered different from *gong.*
qigong	A general term referring to a form of ancient Chinese cultivation practice that involves gentle physical exercises and meditation.
Ren	Forbearance, tolerance, endurance, patience, self-control, restraint, and/or perseverance. It is one of the three principles of Falun Gong.

Shan	Benevolence, compassion, or kindness, one of the three principles of Falun Gong and traditionally emphasized in Buddhist practice.
Shifu	Master or Teacher, a respectful way to address a teacher in traditional Chinese culture.
tai chi	A form of traditional Chinese exercises involving slow, gentle, rhythmic movements that improve *qi,* or vital energy.
wuwei	Non-action, inaction, or without intention
xinxing	Heart-mind nature or moral character. It involves letting go of attachments, enduring hardships, cultivating compassion and forbearance, gaining insight, and elevating moral character.
xiulian	A Chinese term for cultivation: *xiu* means repair, restore, or fix, while *lian* means to improve or refine.
yuanfen	Predestined relationship
Zhen	Truthfulness, one of the three principles of Falun Gong and traditionally emphasized in Taoist practice.
Zhen-Shan-Ren	Truthfulness-compassion-forbearance, the three principles of Falun Gong teachings.

236

References

Note: Due to the time that has passed since the original dissertation, some links may now need to be accessed via the Internet Archive https://web.archive.org/

Ackerman, S. E. (2005). Falun Dafa and the new age movement in Malaysia: Signs of health, symbols of salvation. *Social Compass, 52*(4), 495–511. https://doi.org/10.1177/0037768605058186

Ader, R. (1980). Psychosomatic and psychoimmunologic research. *Psychosomatic Medicine, 42*(3), 307–321. https://doi.org/10.1097/00006842-198005000-00001

Ai, A. L. (2003). Assessing mental health in clinical study on qigong: Between scientific investigation and holistic perspectives. *Seminars in Integrative Medicine, 1*(2), 112–121. https://doi.org/10.1016/S1543-1150(03)00022-X

Ardell, D. (1986). *High Level Wellness: An alternative to doctors, drugs and disease.* Ten Speed Press.

Astin, J. A. (1998). Why patients use alternative medicine: Results of a national study. *Journal of American Medical Association, 279*(19), 1548–1553. https://doi.org/10.1001/jama.279.19.1548

Atkinson, N. L., & Permuth-Levine, R. (2009). Benefits, barriers, and cues to action of yoga practice: A focus group approach. *American Journal of Health Behavior, 33*(1), 3–14. https://doi.org/10.5993/AJHB.33.1.1

Atwood, J. D., & Maltin, L. (1991). Putting Eastern philosophies into Western psychotherapies. *American Journal of Psychotherapy, 45*(3), 368–382. https://doi.org/10.1176/appi.psychotherapy.1991.45.3.368

Australian Bureau of Statistics, & Statistics New Zealand. (2006). ANZSCO: Australian & New Zealand standard classification of occupations. https://www.abs.gov.au/AUSSTATS/abs@.nsf/Lookup/1220.0Main+Features12006

Author Unknown. (1998). Falun Dafa has great effects on improving health status: Survey of over 6,000 cultivators. Retrieved March 3, 2004, from http://www.clearwisdom.net/eng/science_eng/healthsurvey_dalian.html

Author Unknown. (2001). Wellness–The better you. Retrieved July 20, 2020 from https://web.archive.org/web/20071212055611/http://www.pureinsight.org/pi/index.php?news=160

Author Unknown. (2002). Summary of health surveys conducted in mainland China to assess Falun Gong's effects on healing illness and maintaining fitness. Retrieved March 13, 2002, from http://www.pureinsight.org/node/841

Author Unknown. (2003). Russia: Report on the healing effects of Falun Gong from the Moscow business committee. Retrieved April 1, 2003, from http://clearharmony.net/articles/200302/10494.html

Author Unknown. (2008). About the SF-36 (Medical College of Wisconsin.) http://www.mcw.edu/midas/health/SF-36.html

Author Unknown. (2009a). The health benefits of Tai Chi. *Harvard Women's Health Watch, 16*, 2–4. https://www.health.harvard.edu/healthbeat/HB_web/the-health-benefits-of-tai-chi.htm

Author Unknown. (2009b). Yoga for anxiety and depression. *Harvard Mental Health Letter, 25*, 4–5. https://www.health.harvard.edu/mind-and-mood/yoga-for-anxiety-and-depression

Author Unknown (Ed.). (1911). *The melody of the heart* (6th ed.). Simpkin, Marshall, Hamilton, Kent and Co. Ltd.

Authors Unknown. (1999). Summary of results from the 1999 health survey of Falun Gong practitioners in North America. http://www.pureinsight.org/node/1533

Authors Unknown. (2002). Summary of health surveys conducted in mainland China to assess Falun Gong's effects on healing illness and maintaining fitness. Retrieved March 13, 2002, from http://www.pureinsight.org/node/841

Authors Unknown. (2003a). Report on 235 cases of a Falun Gong health survey in North America. Retrieved March 3, 2004, from http://www.clearwisdom.net/emh/articles/2003/3/31/33996.html

Authors Unknown. (2003b). Research report from Taiwan illustrates the power of Falun Gong in improving physical and emotional health while reducing health care expenses. http://www.clearwisdom.net/emh/articles/2003/1/1/30401.html

Barker, C., Pistrang, N., & Elliot, R. (2005). Self-report methods. In *Research methods in clinical psychology* (2nd ed.) (pp. 94–118). http://doi.org/10.1002/0470013435.ch6

Barnes, P. M., Powell-Griner, E., McFann, K., & Nahin, R. L. (2004). Complementary and alternative medicine use among adults: United States, 2002. *Seminars in Integrative Medicine, 2*(2), 54–71. https://doi.org/10.1016/j.sigm.2004.07.003

Bedard, M., Felteau, M., Mazmanian, D., Fedyk, K., Klein, R., Richardson, J., et al. (2003). Pilot evaluation of a mindfulness-based intervention to improve quality of life among individuals who sustained traumatic brain injuries. *Disability and*

Rehabilitation: An International Multidisciplinary Journal, 25(13), 722–731. http://doi.org/10.1080/0963828031000090489

Bishop, F. L., & Lewith, G. T. (2008). Who uses CAM? A narrative review of demographic characteristics and health factors associated with CAM use. *Evidence-based Complementary and Alternative Medicine: eCAM, 7*(1), 11–28. https://doi.org/10.1093/ecam/nen023

Bogart, G. (1991). The use of meditation in psychotherapy: A review of the literature. *American Journal of Psychotherapy, 45*(3), 383–412. https://doi.org/10.1176/appi.psychotherapy.1991.45.3.383

Booth-Kewley, S., Larson, G. E., & Miyoshi, D. K. (2007). Social desirability effects on computerized and paper-and-pencil questionnaires. *Computers in Human Behavior, 23*(1), 463–377. https://doi.org/10.1016/j.chb.2004.10.020

Braithwaite, R. L., Griffin, J., James P., Stephens, T., Murphy, F., & Marrow, T. (1998). Perceived exercise barriers and participation in Tai Chi for elderly African Americans. *American Journal of Health Studies, 14*(4), 169–176.

Brazier, J. E., Harper, R., Jones, N. M., O'Cathain, A., Thomas, K. J., Usherwood, T., et al. (1992). Validating the SF-36 health survey questionnaire: New outcome measure for primary care. *British Medical Journal, 305*(6846), 160¬–164. https://doi.org/10.1136/bmj.305.6846.160

Brooks, J. S., & Scarano, T. (1985). Transcendental Meditation in the treatment of post-Vietnam adjustment. *Journal of Counseling & Development, 64*(3), 212–215. https://doi.org/10.1002/j.1556-6676.1985.tb01078.x

Bruseker, G. (2000). *Falun Gong: A modern Chinese folk Buddhist movement in crisis.* [Unpublished honor's thesis]. The University of Alberta.

Burgdoff, C. A. (2003). How Falun Gong undermines Li Hongzhi's total rhetoric. *Nova Religio: The Journal of Alternative and Emergent Religions, 6*(2), 332–347. https://doi.org/10.1525/nr.2003.6.2.332

Carlson, L. E., Speca, M., Patel, K. D., & Faris, P. (2007). One year pre-post intervention follow-up of psychological, immune, endocrine and blood pressure outcomes of mindfulness-based stress reduction (MBSR) in breast and prostate cancer outpatients. *Brain, Behavior, and Immunity, 21*(8), 1038–1049. https://doi.org/10.1016/j.bbi.2007.04.002

Carlson, L. E., Ursuliak, Z., Goodey, E., Angeen, M., & Speca, M. (2001). The effects of a Mindfulness Meditation-based Stress Reduction program on mood and symptoms of stress in cancer outpatients: 6-month follow-up. *Support Care Cancer, 9*, 112–123. https://doi.org/10.1007/s005200000206

Carpenter, J. T. (1977). Meditation, esoteric traditions: Contributions to psychotherapy. *American Journal of Psychotherapy, 31*(3), 394–404. https://doi.org/10.1176/appi. psychotherapy.1977.31.3.394

Carson, J. W., Carson, K. M., Porter, L. S., Keefe, F. J., Shaw, H., & Miller, J. M. (2007). Yoga for women with metastatic breast cancer: Results from a pilot study. *Journal of Pain and Symptom Management, 33*(3), 331–341. https://doi.org/10.1016/j. jpainsymman.2006.08.009

Chambers, R., Gullone, E., & Allen, N. B. (2009). Mindful emotion regulation: An integrative review. *Clinical Psychology Review 29*(6), 560–572. https://doi. org/10.1016/j.cpr.2009.06.005

Chen, K. (2000). Chinese qigong and the qigong-induced mental disorders. https:// www.bmj.com/rapid-response/2011/10/28/chinese-qigong-and-qigong-induced- mental-disorders

Chen, K., Chen, M., Chao, H., Hung, H., Lin, H., & Li, C. (2009). Sleep quality, depression state, and health status of older adults after silver yoga exercises: Cluster randomized trial. *International Journal of Nursing Studies, 46*(2), 154–163. https://doi.org/10.1016/j.ijnurstu.2008.09.005

Chiesa, A., & Serretti, A. (2009). Mindfulness-based stress reduction for stress management in healthy people: A review and meta-analysis. *The Journal of Alternative and Complementary Medicine, 15*(5), 593–600. http://doi.org/10.1089/ acm.2008.0495

Chiesa, M., & Hobbs, S. (2008). Making sense of social research: How useful is the Hawthorne Effect? *European Journal of Social Psychology, 38*(1), 67–74. https:// doi.org/10.1002/ejsp.401

Christopher, J. C., Christopher, S. E., Dunnagan, T., & Schure, M. (2006). Teaching self-care through mindfulness practices: The application of yoga, meditation, and qigong to counselor training. *Journal of Humanistic Psychology, 46*(4), 494–509. https://doi.org/10.1177/0022167806290215

Clearwisdom editors. (2004). The essentials to sending forth righteous thoughts and the schedule for sending forth righteous thoughts. Retrieved March 2, 2008 from http://www.clearwisdom.net/emh/articles/2004/10/20/53645.html

Clearwisdom editors (Ed.). (2006). *Hearts and minds uplifted: The power of Falun Dafa* (1st ed.). Broad Press International Co. Ltd.

Coruh, B., Ayele, H., Pugh, M., & Mulligan, T. (2005). Does religious activity improve health outcomes? A critical review of the recent literature. *The Journal of Science and Healing, 1*(3), 186–191. https://doi.org/10.1016/j.explore.2005.02.001

Court, J. (2007). Personal communication: Interactions among individuals in specific communities. In M. M. Lau (Ed.). Adelaide, South Australia.

Cowen, V. S., & Adams, T. B. (2005). Physical and perceptual benefits of yoga asana practice: results of a pilot study. *Journal of Bodywork and Movement Therapies, 9*(3), 211–219. https://doi.org/10.1016/j.jbmt.2004.08.001

Cowen, V. S., & Adams, T. B. (2007). Heart rate in yoga asana practice: A comparison of styles. *Journal of Bodywork and Movement Therapies, 11*(1), 91–95. https://doi.org/10.1016/j.jbmt.2006.08.001

Crombie, W. J. (2002, April 18). Meditation changes temperatures: Mind control body in extreme experiments. *Harvard University Gazette,* 1–4. https://news.harvard.edu/gazette/story/2002/04/meditation-changes-temperatures/

Culp, L. K. (Ed.). (n.d.). *Falun Gong Stories: A journey to enlightenment.* Golden Lotus Press.

Cumming, R. G., Voukelatos, A., Lord, S. R., & Rissel, C. (2008). Response letter to Dr. Katz. *Journal of the American Geriatrics Society, 56*(4), 777.

D'Souza, R. (2007). The importance of spirituality in medicine and its application to clinical practice. *The Medical Journal of Australia, 186*(10), S57–S59. https://doi.org/10.5694/j.1326-5377.2007.tb01043.x

Dan, L., Pu, R., Li, F., Li, N., Wang, Q., Lu, Y., et al. (1998). Falun Gong health effect survey of ten-thousand cases in Beijing. Retrieved January 12, 2001, from http://www.clearwisdom.net/eng/science_eng/survey98_1eng.htm

Danhauer, S. C., Mihalko, S. L., Russell, G. B., Campbell, C. R., Felder, L., Daley, K., et al. (2009). Restorative yoga for women with breast cancer: Findings from a randomized pilot study. *Psycho-Oncology, 18,* 360–368. https://doi.org/10.1002/pon.1503

Davidson, R. J., Kabat-Zinn, J., Schmumacher, J., Rosenkranz, M., Muller, D., Santorelli, S. F., et al. (2003). Alterations in brain and immune function produced by Mindfulness Meditation. *Psychosomatic Medicine, 65*(4), 564–570. https://doi.org/10.1097/01.psy.0000077505.67574.e3

Delmonte, M. M. (1984). Psychometric scores and meditation practice: A literature review. *Personality and Individual Differences, 5*(5), 559–563. https://doi.org/10.1016/0191-8869(84)90030-8

Delmonte, M. M. (1985). Meditation and anxiety reduction: A literature review. *Clinical Psychology Review, 5*(2), 91-102. https://doi.org/10.1016/0272-7358(85)90016-9

Derezotes, D. (2000). Evaluation of yoga and meditation trainings with adolescent sex offenders. *Child and Adolescent Social Work, 17*(2), 97–113. https://doi.org/10.1023/A:1007506206353

Donaldson, S. I., & Grant-Vallone, E. J. (2002). Understanding self-report bias in organizational behavior research. *Journal of Business and Psychology, 17*(2), 245-260. https://doi.org/10.1023/A:1019637632584

Easton, M. (2005, Spring). What makes us happy? *University of Toronto Magazine, 32,* 20-26.

Egan, G. (1990). *The skilled helper: A systematic approach to effective helping* (4th ed.). Brooks/Cole Publishing Company.

Eisenberg, D. M., Davis, R. B., Ettner, S. L., Appel, S., Wilkey, S., Van Rompay, M., et al. (1998). Trends in alternative medicine use in the United States, 1990-1997: Results of a follow-up national survey. *Journal of American Medical Association, 280*(18), 1569-1575. https://doi.org/10.1001/jama.280.18.1569

Elliott, R., & Freire, E. (2007). Classical person-centered and experiential perspectives on Rogers (1957). *Psychotherapy: Theory, Research, Practice, Training, 44*(3), 285–288. https://doi.org/10.1037/0033-3204.44.3.285

Emavardhana, T., & Tori, C. D. (1997). Changes in self-concept, ego defense mechanism, and religiosity following seven-day Vipassana Meditation retreats. *Journal for the Scientific Study of Religion, 36*(2), 194–206. https://doi.org/10.2307/1387552

Fadiman, J., & Frager, R. (1994). *Personality and personal growth* (3rd ed.). HarperCollins College Publishers.

Falun Dafa Association. (2009a). Falun Dafa: Frequently asked questions. Retrieved February 26, 2009, from http://www.falundafa.org/eng/faqs.html

Falun Dafa Association. (2009b). Introduction to Falun Dafa. Retrieved February 26, 2009, from http://www.falundafa.org/eng/intro.html

Falun Dafa Information Center. (2008). Overview of Falun Gong. https://faluninfo.net/

Faneuli, N. (1997). The spirituality of wellness. *American Fitness, 15*(6), 42–46.

Fredrickson, B. L. (2000). Cultivating positive emotion to optimize health and well-being. *Prevention and Treatment, 3,* 1–24. https://doi.org/10.1037/1522-3736.3.1.31a

Frost, R. (1969). *The poetry of Robert Frost: The collected poems, complete and unabridged.* Henry Holt and Company, Inc.

Galantino, M. L. (2003). Influence of yoga, walking, and mindfulness meditation on fatigue and body mass index in women living with breast cancer. *Seminars in Integrative Medicine, 1*(3), 151–157. https://doi.org/10.1016/S1543-1150(03)00029-2

Gale, D. D., & Gorman-Yao, W. M. (2003). Falungong: Recent developments in Chinese notions of healing. *Journal of Cultural Diversity, 10*(4), 124–127.

Galli, V. (2002). Our current understanding of psychiatric disorders based on the study of Falun Dafa. https://www.pureinsight.org/node/780

Gallup Jr., G. H. (2002). Why are women more religious? Retrieved August 16, 2009, from http://www.gallup.com/poll/7432/Why-Women-More-Religious.aspx

Garratt, A. M., Ruta, D. A., Abdalla, M. I., Buckingham, J. K., & Russell, I. T. (1993). The SF 36 health survey questionnaire: an outcome measure suitable for routine use within the NHS? *British Medical Journal, 306,* 1440–1444. https://doi.org/10.1136/bmj.306.6890.1440

Girodo, M. (1974). Yoga meditation and flooding in the treatment of anxiety neurosis. *Journal of Behavior Therapy and Experimental Psychiatry, 5*(2), 157–160. https://doi.org/10.1016/0005-7916(74)90104-9

Goldberg, R. J. (1982). Anxiety reduction by self-regulation: Theory, pactice, and evaluation. *Annals of Internal Medicine, 96*(4), 483–487. https://doi.org/10.7326/0003-4819-96-4-483

Goleman, D. (1976). Meditation and consciousness: An Asian approach to mental health. *American Journal of Psychotherapy, 30*(1), 41–54. https://doi.org/10.1176/appi.psychotherapy.1976.30.1.41

Goleman, D., & Gurin, J. (1993). Mind/body medicine-At last. *Psychology Today, 26*(2), 16–18. http://eqi.org/gole7.htm

Gordon, J. S., & Edwards, D. M. (2005). Mind body spirit medicine. *Seminars in Oncology Nursing, 21*(3), 154–158. https://doi.org/10.1016/j.soncn.2005.04.002

Graneheim, U. H., & Lundman, B. (2004). Qualitative content analysis in nursing research: Concepts, procedures and measures to achieve trustworthiness. *Nurse Education Today, 24,* 105–112. https://doi.org/10.1016/j.nedt.2003.10.001

Gross, C. R., Kreitzer, M. J., Rellly-Spong, M., Winbush, N. Y., Schomaker, E. K., & Thomas, W. (2009). Mindfulness meditation training to reduce symptom distress in transplant patients: Rationale, design, and experience with a recycled waitlist. *Clinical Trials, 6*(1), 76–89.

Grossman, P., Niemann, L., Schmidt, S., & Walach, H. (2004). Mindfulness-based stress reduction and health benefits: A meta-analysis. *Journal of Psychosomatic Research, 57*(1), 35–43. https://doi.org/10.1016/S0022-3999(03)00573-7

H.R. Watch, H. R. W. (2002). *Dangerous Meditation: China's Campaign Against Falungong.* Human Rights Watch.

Hadley, R. G., & Mitchell, L. K. (1995). *Counseling research and program evaluation.* Brookes/Cole Publishing Company.

Hanson, W. E., Creswell, J. W., Clark, V. L. P., Petska, K. S., & Creswell, J. D. (2005). Mixed methods research designs in counseling psychology. *Journal of Counseling Psychology, 52*(2), 224–235. http://dx.doi.org/10.1037/0022-0167.52.2.224

Hattie, J. A., Myers, J. E., & Sweeney, T. J. (2004). A factor structure of wellness: Theory, assessment, analysis, and practice. *Journal of Counseling & Development, 82*(3), 354–364. https://doi.org/10.1002/j.1556-6678.2004.tb00321.x

Haynes, A., Hilbers, J., Kivikko, J., & Ratnavuyha, D. (2007). Spirituality and religion in health care practice: A person-centred resource for staff at the Prince of Wales Hospital. SESIAHS, Sydney, Australia.

Heerwegh, D. (2009). Mode differences between face-to-face and web surveys: An experimental investigation of data quality and social desirability effects. *International Journal of Public Opinion Research, 21*(1), 111–121. https://doi.org/10.1093/ijpor/edn054

Heppner, P. P., Kivlighan, J., Dennis M., & Wampold, B. E. (1999). *Research design in counselling* (2nd ed.). Wadsworth Publishing Company.

Hilbers, J., Haynes, A., Kivikko, J., & Ratnavuyha, D. (2007). Spirituality/Religion and health: Research report (Phase two). SESIAHS, Sydney.

Hindle, T. (2008). The Hawthorne Effect. *Guide to Management Ideas & Gurus,* 99-100.

Hogan, M. (2005). Physical and cognitive activity and exercise for older adults: A review. *International Journal of Aging & Human Development, 60*(2), 95–126. https://doi.org/10.2190/PTG9-XDVM-YETA-MKXA

Howatt, W. A. (2000). *The human services counseling toolbox.* Cengage Learning.

Hsia Chang, M. (2004). *Falun Gong: The end of days.* Yale University Press.

Hu, P. (2003). The Falungong phenomenon. *China Watch Forum, 4,* 11–27.

Irons, E. (2003). Falun Gong and the sectarian religion paradigm. *Nova Religio: The Journal of Alternative and Emergent Religions, 6*(2), 244–262. https://doi.org/10.1525/nr.2003.6.2.244

Irwin, M. R., Olmstead, R., & Oxman, M. N. (2007). Augmenting immune responses to varicella-zoster virus in older adults: A randomized, controlled trial of Tai Chi. *Journal of the American Geriatrics Society, 55*(4), 511–517. https://doi.org/10.1111/j.1532-5415.2007.01109.x

Irwin, M. R., Pike, J. L., Cole, J. C., & Oxman, M. N. (2003). Effects of a behavioral intervention, Tai Chi Chih, on varicella-zoster virus specific immunity and health functioning in older adults. *Psychosomatic Medicine, 65*(5), 824–830. https://doi.org/10.1097/01.PSY.0000088591.86103.8F

Jacobs, A. (2009, 27 April 2009). China still presses crusade against Falun Gong. *The New York Times.*

Jacobs, G. D. (2001). The physiology of mind–body interactions: The stress response and the relaxation response. *Journal of Alternative and Complementary Medicine, 7*(Supplement 1), S-83–S-92. https://doi.org/10.1089/107555301753393841

James, R. K., & Gilliland, R. K. (2008). *Crisis intervention strategies* (6th ed.). Thomson Brooks/Cole Publishing Co.

Jang, H.-S., & Lee, M. S. (2004). Effects of Qi therapy (external qigong) on premenstrual syndrome: A randomized placebo-controlled study. *Journal of Alternative & Complementary Medicine, 10*(3), 456–462. https://doi.org/10.1089/1075553041323902

Jang, H.-S., Lee, M. S., Kim, M.-J., & Chong, E. S. (2004). Effects of Qi-therapy on premenstrual dyndrome. *International Journal of Neuroscience, 114*(8), 909–921. https://doi.org/10.1080/00207450490450163

Javnbakhta, M., Kenari, R. H., & Ghasemi, M. (2009). Effects of yoga on depression and anxiety of women. *Complementary Therapies in Clinical Practice, 15*(2), 102–104. https://doi.org/10.1016/j.ctcp.2009.01.003

Jayadevappa, R., Johnson, J. C., Bloom, B. S., Nidich, S., Desai, S., Chhatre, S., et al. (2007). Effectiveness of Transcendental Meditation on functional capacity and quality of life of African Americans with congestive heart failure: A randomized control study. *National Institutes of Health Public Access, US, 17,* 72–77. http://www.pubmedcentral.nih.gov/articlerender.fcgi?artid=2048830

Jenkinson, C., Coulter, A., & Wright, L. (1993). Short form 36 (SF-36) health survey questionnaire: Normative data for adults of working age. *British Medical Journal, 306*(6890), 1437–1440. https://doi.org/10.1136/bmj.306.6890.1437

Johansson, M., Hassmen, P., & Jouper, J. (2008). Acute effects of qigong exercise on mood and anxiety. *International Journal of Stress Management, 15*(2), 199–207. https://doi.org/10.1037/1072-5245.15.2.199.

Johnson, S. S., & Kushner, R. F. (2001). Mindbody medicine: An introduction for the generalist physician and nutritionist. *Nutrition in Clinical Care, 4*(5), 256–264. https://doi.org/10.1046/j.1523-5408.2001.00006.x

Kakigi, R., Nakata, H., Inui, K., Hiroe, N., Nagata, O., Honda, M., et al. (2005). Intracerebral pain processing in a yoga master who claims not to feel pain during meditation. *European Journal of Pain, 9*(5), 581–589. https://doi.org/10.1016/j.ejpain.2004.12.006

Kang, Y. S., Choi, S. Y., & Ryu, E. (2009). The effectiveness of a stress coping program based on mindfulness meditation on the stress, anxiety, and depression experienced by nursing students in Korea. *Nurse Education Today, 29*(5), 538–543. https://doi.org/10.1016/j.nedt.2008.12.003

Katz, A. R. (2008). Reduced falls in the elderly: Tai chi or placebo or Hawthorne effect? *Journal of the American Geriatrics Society, 56*(4), 776–777. https://doi.org/10.1111/j.1532-5415.2008.01651.x

Keefer, L., & Blanchard, E. B. (2002). A one year follow-up of relaxation response meditation as a treatment for irritable bowel syndrome. *Behaviour Research and Therapy, 40*(5), 541–546. https://doi.org/10.1016/S0005-7967(01)00065-1

Kessler, R. C., Davis, R. B., Foster, D. F., Van Rompay, M. I., Walters, E. E., Wilkey, S. A., et al. (2001). Long-term trends in the use of complementary and alternative medical therapies in the United States. *Annals of Internal Medicine 135*(4), 262–268. https://doi.org/10.7326/0003-4819-135-4-200108210-00011

Khalsa, H. K. (2003). Yoga: an adjunct to infertility treatment. *Sexuality, Reproduction and Menopause, 1*(1), 46–51. https://doi.org/10.1016/j.sram.2004.02.024

Khalsa, H. K. (2004). How yoga, meditation, and a yogic lifestyle can help women meet the challenges of perimenopause and menopause. *Sexuality, Reproduction and Menopause, 2*(3), 169–175. https://doi.org/10.1016/j.sram.2004.07.011

Kirkland, R. (1998). Neiye: Inner Cultivation. https://faculty.franklin.uga.edu/kirkland/sites/faculty.franklin.uga.edu.kirkland/files/NEIYEH98.pdf

Kirkland, R. (2005). *Taoism: The Enduring Tradition* (2nd ed.). Routledge.

Kjaer, T. W., Bertelsen, C., Piccini, P., Brooks, D., Alving, J., & Lou, H. C. (2002). Increased dopamine tone during meditation-induced change of consciousness. *Cognitive Brain Research, 13*(2), 255–259. https://doi.org/10.1016/S0926-6410(01)00106-9

Koenig, H. G. (1999). *The healing power of faith: Science explores medicine's last great frontier.* Simon & Schuster.

Koenig, H. G. (2004a). Religion, spirituality, and medicine: Research findings and implications for clinical practice. *Southern Medical Association, 97*(12), 1194–1200. https://doi.org/10.1097/01.SMJ.0000146489.21837.CE

Koenig, H. G. (2004b). Spirituality, wellness, and quality of Life. *Sexuality, Reproduction & Menopause, 2*(2), 76–82. https://doi.org/10.1016/j.sram.2004.04.004

Koenig, H. G. (2007). Religion, spirituality and medicine in Australia: Research and clinical practice. *The Medical Journal of Australia, 186*, S45–S46. https://doi.org/10.5694/j.1326-5377.2007.tb01039.x

Koenig, H. G., & Cohen, H. J. (Eds.). (2002). *The link between religion and health: Psychoneuroimmunology and the faith factor.* Oxford University Press.

Koenig, H. G., E., M. M., & Larson, D. B. (2001). *Handbook of religion and health.* Oxford University Press.

Krisanaprakornkit, T., C., Krisanaprakornkit, W., & Piyavhatkul, N. (2007). Meditation therapies for attention deficit/hyperactivity disorder (Protocol). *Cochrane Database of Systematic Reviews 2007*(2), Art. No.: CD006507.

Krisanaprakornkit, T., Krisanaprakornkit, W., Piyavhatkul, N., & Laopaiboon, M. (2006). Meditation therapy for anxiety disorders. *Cochrane Database of Systematic Reviews 2006*(1), Art. No.: CD004998.

Kuentzel, J. G., Henderson, M. J., & Melville, C. L. (2008). The impact of social desirability biases on self-report among college student and problem gamblers. *Journal of Gambling Studies, 24*(3), 307–319. https://doi.org/10.1007/s10899-008-9094-8

Kutolowski, M. (2007). Transcending the mundane. Retrieved October 31, 2009 from https://faluninfo.net/transcending-the-mundane/

Laselle, K. M., & Russell, T. T. (1993). To what extent are school counselors using meditation and relaxation techniques? *School Counselor, 40*(3), 178–183. https://www.jstor.com/stable/23901514

Lau, M. M. (2001). *Exploring counselors' burnout and alternative coping strategies: Falun Dafa as an alternative coping strategy.* [Unpublished master's case study]. The University of South Australia.

Lazar, S. W., Kerr, C. E., Wasserman, R. H., Gray, J. R., Greve, D. N., Treadway, M. T., et al. (2005). Meditation experience is associated with increased cortical thickness. *NeuroReport, 16*(17), 1893–1897. https://doi.org/10.1097/01.wnr.0000186598.66243.19

Lee, M. M., Lin, S. S., Wrensch, M. R., Adler, S. R., & Eisenberg, D. (2000). Alternative therapies used by women with breast cancer in four ethnic populations. *Journal of the National Cancer Institute, 92*(1), 42–47. https://doi.org/10.1093/jnci/92.1.42

Lee, M. S., Huh, H. J., Kim, B. G., Ryu, H., Lee, H.-S., Kim, J.-M., et al. (2002). Effects of Qi-training on heart rate variability. *American Journal of Chinese Medicine, 30*(4), 463–470. https://doi.org/10.1142/S0192415X02000491

Lee, M. S., & Jang, H. S. (2005). Two case reports of the acute effects of Qi therapy (external qigong) on symptoms of cancer: Short report. *Complementary Therapies in Clinical Practice, 11*(3), 211–213. https://doi.org/10.1016/j.ctcp.2005.01.002

Lee, M. S., Jeong, S. M., Jang, H. S., Ryu, H., & Moon, S. R. (2003). Effects of in vitro and in vivo Qi-therapy on neutrophil superoxide generation in healthy male subjects. *American Journal of Chinese Medicine, 31*(4), 623–628. https://doi.org/10.1142/S0192415X03001119

Lee, M. S., Kang, C. W., Ryu, H., & Moon, S. R. (2004). Endocrine and immune effects of Qi-training. *International Journal of Neuroscience, 114*(4), 529–537. https://doi.org/10.1080/00207450490422849

Lee, M. S., & Ryu, H. (2004). QI-training enhances neutrophil function by increasing growth hormone levels in elderly men. *International Journal of Neuroscience, 114*(10), 1313–1322. https://doi.org/10.1080/00207450490476084

Lee, M. S., Ryu, H., Song, J., & Moon, S. R. (2004). Brief communication: Effects of Qi-training (qigong) on forearm blood gas concentrations. *International Journal of Neuroscience, 114*(1 1), 1503–1510.

Lemonick, M. D. (2005, January 17). The biology of joy. *Time Magazine, 165*, 50-53.

Leung, Y., & Singhal, A. (2004). An examination of the relationship between qigong meditation and personality. *Social Behavior & Personality, 32*(4), 313–320. https://doi.org/10.2224/sbp.2004.32.4.313

Li, F., Duncan, T. E., Duncan, S. C., McAuley, E., Chaumeton, N. R., & Harmer, P. (2001). Enhancing the psychological well-being of elderly individuals through Tai Chi exercise: A latent growth curve analysis. *Structural Equation Modeling, 8*(1), 53–83. https://doi.org/10.1207/S15328007SEM0801_4

Li, F., McAuley, E., Harmer, P., Duncan, T. E., & Chaumeton, N. R. (2001). Tai Chi enhances self-efficacy and exercise behavior in older adults. *Journal of Aging and Physical Activity, 9*(2), 161–171. https://doi.org/10.1123/japa.9.2.161

Li, H. (1996). Fa-teaching given at the Conference in Sydney. Falun Dafa Experience Sharing Conference. https://en.falundafa.org/eng/lectures/1996L_2018.html

Li, H. (1999). Teaching the Fa at Fa Conference in Australia. Falun Dafa Experience Sharing Conference. https://en.falundafa.org/eng/lectures/19990502L.html

Li, H. (2001a). *Falun Gong.* Fair Winds Press.

Li, H. (2001b). *Zhuan Falun.* Fair Winds Press.

Li, H. (2002). Righteous Thoughts. Retrieved May 30, 2008, from http://en.minghui.org/html/articles/2002/10/14/27578.html

Li, H. (2003). *Zhuan Falun: Turning the law wheel* (English Draft Translation Edition, North America ed.). Yih Chyun Book Corp.

Li, H. (2007a). *Fa teaching at the 2007 New York Fa Conference.* Falun Dafa Experience Sharing Conference. https://en.falundafa.org/eng/lectures/20070407L.html

Li, H. (2007b). *Fa teaching at the U.S. Capital, Washington D.C.* Falun Dafa Experience Sharing Conference. https://en.falundafa.org/eng/lectures/20070722L.html

Li, H. (2008). *Fa teaching at the 2008 New York conference.* Falun Dafa Experience Sharing Conference. https://en.minghui.org/emh/articles/2008/6/22/98383.html

Li, M., Chen, K., & Mo, Z. (2002). Use of qigong therapy in the detoxification of heroin addicts. *Alternative Therapies, 8*(1), 50–59.

Li, Q., Li, P., Garcia, G. E., Johnson, R. J., & Feng, L. (2005). Genomic profiling of neutrophil transcripts in Asian Qigong practitioners: A pilot study in gene regulation by mind-body interaction. *Journal of Alternative and Complementary Medicine, 11*(1), 29–39. https://doi.org/10.1089/acm.2005.11.29

Life and hope renewed (2005). *The healing power of Falun Dafa.*. Yih Chyun Corp.

Lindberg, D. A. (2005). Integrative review of research related to meditation, spirituality, and the elderly. *Geriatric Nursing 26*(6), 372–377. https://doi.org/10.1016/j.gerinurse.2005.09.013

Lio, M., Hu, Y., He, M., Huang, L., Chen, L., & Cheng, S. (2003). The effect of practicing qigong on health status: A case study of Falun Dafa practitioners in Taiwan. [Unpublished research]. National Taiwan University.

Long, L., Huntley, A., & Ernst, E. (2001). Which complementary and alternative therapies benefit which conditions? A survey of the opinions of 223 professional organizations. *Complementary Therapies in Medicine, 9*(3), 178–185. https://doi.org/10.1054/ctim.2001.0453

Lowe, S. (2003). Chinese and international contexts for the rise of Falun Gong. *Nova Religio: The Journal of Alternative and Emergent Religions, 6*(2), 263–276. https://doi.org/10.1525/nr.2003.6.2.263

Maciocia, G. (1989). *The foundations of Chinese medicine.* Churchill Livingston.

Madsen, R. (2000). Understanding Falun Gong. *Current History: A Journal of Contemporary World Affairs, 99*(638), 243–247.

Mamtani, R., & Cimino, A. (2002). A primer of complementary and alternative medicine and its relevance in the treatment of mental health problems. *Psychiatric Quarterly, 73*(4), 367–381. https://doi.org/10.1023/A:1020472218839

Manocha, R. (2000). Why meditation? *Australian Family Physician, 29*(12), 1135–1138.

Mao, J. J., Farrar, J. T., Xie, S. X., Bowman, M. A., & Armstrong, K. (2007). Use of complementary and alternative medicine and prayer among a national sample of cancer survivors compared to other populations without cancer. *Complementary Therapies in Medicine 15*(1), 21–29. https://doi.org/10.1016/j.ctim.2006.07.006

Marlatt, G. A., & Kristeller, J. L. (1999). Mindfulness and meditation. In W. R. Miller (Ed.), *Integrating spirituality into treatment: Resources for practitioners.* (pp. 67–84). American Psychological Association.

Maselko, J., & Kubzansky, L. D. (2006). Gender differences in religious practices, spiritual experiences and health: Results from the U.S. general social survey. *Social Science & Medicine, 62*(11), 2848–2860. https://doi.org/10.1016/j.socscimed.2005.11.008

Matas, D. (2009). *Why Chinese communists repress Falun Gong.* Remarks delivered to an International Conference on Religious Freedom in China, European Parliament, Brussels. http://www.davidkilgour.com/2009/Apr_14_2009_01.php

Matas, D., & Kilgour, D. (2006). Report into allegations of organ harvesting of Falun Gong practitioners in China. Ottawa, Canada.

Matas, D., & Kilgour, D. (2007). *Bloody harvest:* Revised report into allegations of organ harvesting of Falun Gong practitioners in China. Ottawa, Canada.

McCarney, R., Warner, J., Iliffe, S., van Haselen, R., Griffin, M., & Fisher, P. (2007). The Hawthorne Effect: A randomised, controlled trial. *BMC Medical Research Methodology, 7*, 30–38. https://doi.org/10.1186/1471-2288-7-30

McCown, D. (2004). Cognitive and perceptual benefits of meditation. *Seminars in Integrative Medicine, 2*(4), 148–151. https://doi.org/10.1016/j.sigm.2004.12.001

McCoy, W. F., & Zhang, L. (Eds.). (n.d.). *Falun Gong Stories: A journey to ultimate health* (1st ed.). Golden Lotus Press.

McHorney, C. A., Ware, J. E., Lu, R. J. F., & Sherbourne, C. D. (1994). The MOS 36-Item Short-Form Health Survey (SF-36): III. Tests of data quality, scaling assumptions, and reliability across diverse patient groups. *Medical Care, 32*(1), 40–66. http://doi.org/10.1097/00005650-199401000-00004

Mearns, D., & Thorne, B. (2007). *Person-centred counselling in action* (3rd ed.). Sage Publications.

Mehta, D. H., Phillips, R. S., Davis, R. B., & McCarthy, E. P. (2007). Use of complementary and alternative therapies by Asian Americans: Results from the National Health Interview Survey. *Journal of General Internal Medicine, 22*(6), 762–767. https://doi.org/10.1007/s11606-007-0166-8

Merry, T. (2002). *Learning and being in person-centred counselling* (2nd ed.). PCCS Books.

Miles, M. B., & Huberman, A. M. (1994). *Qualitative data analysis: An expanded sourcebook* (2nd ed.). Sage Publications.

Miller, J. J., Fletcher, K., & Kabat-Zinn, J. (1995). Three-year follow-up and clinical implication of a Mindfulness Meditation-based Stress Reduction intervention in the treatment of anxiety disorders. *General Hospital Psychiatry, 17*(3), 192–200. https://doi.org/10.1016/0163-8343(95)00025-M

Monk-Turner, E. (2003). The benefits of meditation: Experimental findings. *The Social Science Journal, 40*(3), 465–470. https://doi.org/10.1016/S0362-3319(03)00043-0

Moreira-Almeida, A., & Koenig, H. G. (2006). Retaining the meaning of the words religiousness and spirituality: A commentary on the WHOQOL SRPB group's "A cross-cultural study of spirituality, religion, and personal beliefs as components of quality of life." *Social Science & Medicine, 63*(4), 843–845. https://doi.org/10.1016/j.socscimed.2006.03.001

Myers, J. E., & Sweeney, T. J. (2005a). The indivisible self: An evidence-based model of wellness. *Journal of Individual Psychology, 61*(3), 269–279.

Myers, J. E., & Sweeney, T. J. (Eds.). (2005b). *Counseling for wellness: Theory, research, and practice.* American Counseling Association.

Myers, J. E., Sweeney, T. J., & Witmer, J. M. (2000). The Wheel of Wellness counseling for wellness: A holistic model for treatment planning. *Journal of Counseling & Development, 78*, 251–266. https://doi.org/10.1002/j.1556-6676.2000.tb01906.x

Naranjo, C., & Ornstein, R. E. (1971). *On the psychology of meditation.* George Allen & Unwin.

NCCAM. (2008, February 2007). What is CAM? NCCAM Publication No. D347. Retrieved May 28, 2008, from http://nccam.nih.gov/health/whatiscam/

NCCAM. (2009). *Tai chi for health purposes.* National Institute of Health. Retrieved April 25, 2009, from http://nccam.nih.gov/health/taichi/

NHMRC. (2007). *National statement on ethical conduct in human research - updated 2018.* National Health and Medical Research Council. https://www.nhmrc.gov.au/about-us/publications/national-statement-ethical-conduct-human-research-2007-updated-2018

North America Dafa disciples. (2003). Report on 235 cases of a Falun Gong health survey in North America. https://en.minghui.org/emh/articles/2003/3/31/33996.html

Northrup, D. A. (1996). The problem of the self-report in survey research. *Institute for Social Research Newsletter, York University, 11*, 2. Retrieved April 30, 2009, from http://www.math.yorku.ca/ISR/self.htm

O'Leary, Z. (2004). Indicators of good research. *In The essential guide to doing research* (pp. 56–65). Sage Publications.

Oh, M. Y., & Ramaprasad, J. (2003). Halo effect: Conceptual definition and empirical exploration with regard to South Korean subsidiaries of U.S. and Japanese multinational corporations. *Journal of Communication Management, 7*(4), 317–332. https://doi.org/10.1108/13632540310807458

Ospina, M. B., Bond, K., Karkhaneh, M., Buscemi, N., Dryden, D. M., Barnes, V., et al. (2008). Clinical trials of meditation practices in health care: Characteristics and quality. *Journal of Alternative & Complementary Medicine, 14*(10), 1199–1213. https://doi.org/10.1089/acm.2008.0307

Ownby, D. (2000, December 20). Falungong as a cultural revitalization movement: An historian looks at contemporary China. *Transnational China Project.* http://www.ruf.rice.edu/~tnchina/commentary/ownby1000.html

Ownby, D. (2001). Falungong and Canada's China policy. *International Journal, 56*(2), 183–204. https://doi.org/10.1177/002070200105600201

Ownby, D. (2003a). A history for Falun Gong: Popular religion and the Chinese state since the Ming Dynasty. *Nova Religio: The Journal of Alternative and Emergent Religions, 6*(2), 223–243. https://doi.org/10.1525/nr.2003.6.2.223

Ownby, D. (2003b). The Falun Gong in the new world. *European Journal of East Asian Studies, 2*(2), 303–320. Retrieved from https://www.jstor.org/stable/i23615133

Ownby, D. (2005). Unofficial religions in China: Beyond the Party's rules–Statement of Professor David Ownby. https://www.cecc.gov/events/roundtables/unofficial-religions-in-china-beyond-the-partys-rules

Ownby, D. (2008a). *Falun Gong and the future of China.* Oxford University Press.

Ownby, D. (2008b). In search of charisma: The Falun Gong diaspora. *Nova Religio: The Journal of Alternative and Emergent Religions, 12*(2), 106–120. https://doi.org/10.1525/nr.2008.12.2.106

Oxford Dictionary (Ed.) (2005) *Oxford dictionary of English* (2nd ed.). In C. Soanes & A. Stevenson (Eds.), Oxford University Press.

Oz, M. C. (2003, January 20). Medical Meditation: Say "Om" before surgery. *Time Magazine, US ed., Special Issue: How your mind can heal your body, 161,* 1-2.

Palmer, D. (2007). *Qigong fever.* New York: Columbia University Press.

Palmer, S. J. (2003). From healing to protest: Conversion patterns among the practitioners of Falun Gong. *Nova Religio: The Journal of Alternative and Emergent Religions, 6*(2), 348–364. https://doi.org/10.1525/nr.2003.6.2.348

Parker, N. (2004). What is Falun Gong? An introduction to the practice and how it developed in China and around the world. *Compassion, 5,* 40–43.

Peach, H. G. (2003). Religion, spirituality and health: How should Australia's medical professionals respond? *The Medical Journal of Australia, 178*(2), 86–88. https://doi.org/10.5694/j.1326-5377.2003.tb05071.x

Pelletier, K. R. (1978). *Mind as healer, mind as slayer: A holistic approach to preventing stress disorders.* George Allen & Unwin.

Pelletier, K. R. (2002). Mind as healer, mind as slayer: Mindbody medicine comes of age [Editorial]. *Advances in Mind-Body Medicine, 18*(1), 4–15.

Penny, B. (2001). *The past, present and future of Falun Gong.* Retrieved May 18, 2008, from http://www.nla.gov.au/grants/haroldwhite/papers/bpenny.html

Penny, B. (2003). The life and times of Li Hongzhi: Falun Gong and religious biography. *The China Quarterly, 175,* 643–661. https://doi.org/10.1017/S0305741003000389

Penny, B. (2005). The Falun Gong, Buddhism and "Buddhist qigong." *Asian Studies Review, 29*(1), 35–46. https://doi.org/10.1080/10357820500139513

Perez-De-Albeniz, A., & Holmes, J. (2000). Meditation: Concepts, effects and uses in therapy. *International Journal of Psychotherapy, 5*(1), 49–58. https://doi.org/10.1080/13569080050020263

Plotinus. (1975). *The essential Plotinus: Representative treatises from the Enneads* (E. J. O'Brien, Trans. 2nd ed.). Hackett Publishing Company, Inc.

Porter, N. (2003). Falun Gong in the United States: An ethnographic study. Dissertation. com. https://scholarcommons.usf.edu/etd/1451/

Porter, N. (2005). Professional practitioners and contact persons: Explicating special types of Falun Gong practitioners. *Nova Religio: The Journal of Alternative and Emergent Religion, 9*(2), 62–83. https://doi.org/10.1525/nr.2005.9.2.062

Prince, S. A., Adamo, K. B., Hamel, M. E., Hardt, J., Connor Gorber, S., & Tremblay, M. (2008). A comparison of direct versus self-report measures for assessing physical activity in adults: A systematic review. *The International Journal of Behavioral Nutrition and Physical Activity, 5,* 56. https://doi.org/10.1186/1479-5868-5-56

Pullen, L. C. (2000). CBS health watch: Three part series on Falun Dafa. http://en.minghui.org/emh/articles/2000/4/17/8467p.html

Razavi, T. (2001). Self-report measures: An overview of concerns and limitations of questionnaire use in occupational stress research. *E-Prints Soton,* University of Southampton. http://eprints.soton.ac.uk/35712/

Reibel, D. K., Greeson, J. M., Brainard, G. C., & Rosenzweig, S. (2001). Mindfulness-based stress reduction and health-related quality of life in a heterogeneous patient population. *General Hospital Psychiatry, 23*(4), 183–192. https://doi.org/10.1016/S0163-8343(01)00149-9

Rippentrop, E. A., Altmaier, E. M., Chen, J. J., Found, E. M., & Keffala, V. J. (2005). The relationship between religion/spirituality and physical health, mental health, and pain in a chronic pain population. *Pain, 116*(3), 311–321. https://doi.org/10.1016/j.pain.2005.05.008

Rogers, C. E., Larkey, L. K., & Keller, C. (2009). A review of clinical trials of Tai Chi and qigong in older adults. *Research Western Journal of Nursing, 31*(2), 245–279. https://doi.org/10.1177/0193945908327529

Rogers, C. R. (1951). *Client-centered therapy: Its current practice, implications, and theory* (1965 paperback ed.). Houghton Mifflin Company.

Rogers, C. R. (1957). The necessary and sufficient conditions of therapeutic personality change. *Journal of Consulting Psychology, 21*(2), 95–103. https://doi.org/10.1037/h0045357

Rosenzweig, S., Greeson, J. M., Reibel, D. K., Green, J. S., Jasser, S. A., & Beasley, D. (2009). Mindfulness-based stress reduction for chronic pain conditions: Variation in treatment outcomes and role of home meditation practice. *Journal of Psychosomatic Research, 68*(1), 29–36. https://doi.org/10.1016/j.jpsychores.2009.03.010

Roth, B., & Robbins, D. (2004). Mindfulness-Based Stress Reduction and health-related quality of life: Findings from a bilingual inner-city patient population. *Psychosomatic Medicine, 66*(1), 113–123. https://doi.org/10.1097/01.PSY.0000097337.00754.09

Sancier, K. M. (1996). Medical applications of qigong. *Alternative Therapies in Health and Medicine, 2*(1), 40–46.

Sancier, K. M. (1999). Therapeutic benefits of qigong exercises in combination with drugs. *Journal of Alternative and Complementary Medicine, 5*(4), 383–389. https://doi.org/10.1089/acm.1999.5.383

Sancier, K. M., & Holman, D. (2004). Commentary: Multifaceted health benefits of medical qigong. *The Journal of Alternative and Complementary Medicine, 10*(1), 163–165. https://doi.org/10.1089/107555304322849084

Sandelowski, M. (2000). Combining qualitative and quantitative sampling, data collection, and analysis techniques in mixed-method studies. *Research in Nursing and Health, 23*(3), 246–255.

Sandlund, E. S., & Norlander, T. (2000). The effects of Tai Chi Chuan relaxation and exercise on stress responses and well-being: An overview of research. *International Journal of Stress Management, 7*(2), 139–149. https://doi.org/10.1023/A:1009536319034

Sattin, R. W., Easley, K. A., Wolf, S. L., Chen, Y., & Kutner, M. H. (2005). Reduction in fear of falling through intense Tai Chi exercise training in older, transitionally frail adults. *Journal of the American Geriatrics Society, 53*(7), 1168–1178. https://doi.org/10.1111/j.1532-5415.2005.53375.x

Schechter, D. (2000). *Falun Gong's challenge to China: Spiritual practice or "evil cult"?* Akashic Books.

Scherer-Dickson, N. (2004). Current developments of metacognitive concepts and their clinical implications: Mindfulness-based cognitive therapy for depression.

Counselling Psychology Quarterly, 17(2), 223–234. https://doi.org/10.1080/0951 5070410001728253

Schopen, A., & Freeman, B. (1992). Meditation: The forgotten Western tradition. *Counseling and Values, 36*(2), 123–134. https://doi.org/10.1002/j.2161-007X.1991. tb00969.x

Schreiner, I., & Malcolm, J. P. (2008). The benefits of mindfulness meditation: Changes in emotional states of depression, anxiety, and stress. *Behaviour Change, 25*(3), 156–168. https://doi.org/10.1375/bech.25.3.156

Schure, M. B., Christopher, J., & Christopher, S. (2008). Mind-body medicine and the art of self-care: Teaching mindfulness to counseling students through yoga, meditation, and Qigong. *Journal of Counseling and Development, 86*(1), 47–56. https://doi.org/10.1002/j.1556-6678.2008.tb00625.x

Schwartz, G. E., Davidson, R. J., & Goleman, D. J. (1978). Patterning of cognitive and somatic processes in the self-regulation of anxiety: Effects of meditation versus exercise. *Psychosomatic Medicine, 40*(4), 321–328.

Selhub, E. (2007). Mind-body medicine for treating depression: Using the mind to alter the body's response to stress. *Alternative and Complementary Therapies, 13*(1), 4–9. https://doi.org/10.1089/act.2007.13107

Shapiro Jr., D. H. (1980). *Meditation: Self-regulation strategy and altered state of consciousness.* Aldine Publishing Company.

Shapiro Jr., D. H. (1992). Adverse effects of meditation: A preliminary investigation of long-term meditators. *International Journal of Psychosomatics, 39*(1–4), 62¬–67.

Shapiro, S. L., Astin, J. A., Bishop, S. R., & Cordova, M. (2005). Mindfulness-Based Stress Reduction for health care professionals: Results from a randomized trial. *International Journal of Stress Management, 12*(2), 164–176. https://doi. org/10.1037/1072-5245.12.2.164

Shapiro, S. L., Schwartz, G. E., & Bonner, G. (1998). Effects of Mindfulness-Based Stress Reduction on medical and premedical students. *Journal of Behavioral Medicine, 21*(6), 581–599. https://doi.org/10.1023/A:1018700829825

Sharif, F., & Masoumi, S. (2005). A qualitative study of nursing student experiences of clinical practice. *BMC Nursing, 4*(6). https://doi.org/10.1186/1472-6955-4-6

Shealy, C. N., Norris, P., & Fahrion, S. L. (2002). *Mind-body medicines. A National Curriculum For Medical Students.* http://www.amsa.org/humed/CAM/resources.cfm

Shorofi, S. A., & Arbon, P. (2009). Complementary and alternative medicine (CAM) among hospitalised patients: An Australian study. *Complementary Therapies in Clinical Practice, 16*(2), 86–91. https://doi.org/10.1016/j.ctcp.2009.09.009

Sierpina, V., Levine, R., Astin, J., & Tan, A. (2007). Use of mind-body therapies in psychiatry and family medicine faculty and residents: Attitudes, barriers, and gender differences. *The Journal of Science and Healing, 3*(2), 129–135. https://doi.org/10.1016/j.explore.2006.12.001

Silverthorn, N. A., & Gekoski, W. L. (1995). Social desirability effects on measures of adjustment to university, independence from parents, and self-efficacy. *Journal of Clinical Psychology, 51*(2), 244–251.

Singer, R. (2006). *Mindfulness meditation in Western society.* Ezinearticles. http://ezinearticles.com/?Mindfulness-Meditation-in-Western-Society&id=228788

Singh, A. N. (2006, April). *Role of yoga therapies in psychosomatic disorders.* Presented at the International Congress Series; Proceedings of the 18th World Congress on Psychosomatic Medicine, 21-26 August 2005, Kobe, Japan. https://doi.org/10.1016/j.ics.2005.11.096

Siti, Z. M., Tahir, A., Farah, I., Ami Fazlin, S. M., Sondi, S., Azman, A. H., et al. (2009). Use of traditional and complementary medicine in Malaysia: A baseline study. *Complementary Therapies in Medicine, 17*(5-6) 292–299. https://doi.org/10.1016/j.ctim.2009.04.002

Skoro-Kondza, L., Tai, S. S., Gadelrab, R., Drincevic, D., & Greenhalgh, T. (2009). Community based yoga classes for type 2 diabetes: An exploratory randomised controlled trial. *BMC Health Services Research, 9*(33). https://doi.org/10.1186/1472-6963-9-33

Smith, B. J., Tang, K., & Nutbeam, D. (2006). WHO health promotion glossary: New terms. *Health Promotion International, 21*(4), 340–345. https://doi.org/10.1093/heapro/dal033

Smith, C., Hancock, H., Blake-Mortimer, J., & Eckert, K. (2007). A randomised comparative trial of yoga and relaxation to reduce stress and anxiety. *Complementary Therapies in Medicine, 15*(2), 77–83. https://doi.org/10.1016/j.ctim.2006.05.001

Speca, M., Carlson, L. E., Goodey, E., & Angeen, M. (2000). A randomized, wait-list controlled clinical trial: The effect of a Mindfulness Meditation-based Stress Reduction program on mood and symptoms of stress in cancer outpatients. *Psychosomatic Medicine, 62*(5), 613–622.

Spector, P. E. (1994). Using self-report questionnaires in OB research: A comment on the use of a controversial method. *Journal of Organizational Behavior, 15*(5), 385–392. https://doi.org/10.1002/job.4030150503

Spiegel, M. (2002). *Dangerous Meditation: China's campaign against Falungong.* Human Rights Watch.

Stanfeld, S. A., Roberts, R., & Foot, S. P. (1997). Assessing the validity of the SF-36 General Health Survey. *Quality of Life Research, 6*(3), 217–224. https://doi.org/10.1023/A:1026406620756

Sumter, M. T., Monk-Turner, E., & Turner, C. (2007). The potential benefits of meditation in a correctional setting. *Corrections Today, 69*(4), 56–67.

Sumter, M. T., Monk-Turner, E., & Turner, C. (2009). The benefits of meditation practice in the correctional setting. *Journal of Correctional Health Care, 15*(1), 47–57. https://doi.org/10.1177/1078345808326621

Swinford, P. A. (1989). An overview. In P. A. Swinford & J. A. Webster (Eds.), *Promoting Wellness: A nurse's handbook* (pp. 302). Aspen Publishers, Inc.

Tacón, A. M., McComb, J., Caldera, Y., & Randolph, P. (2003). Mindfulness meditation, anxiety reduction, and heart disease: A pilot study. *Family and Community Health, 26*(1), 25–33. https://doi.org/10.1097/00003727-200301000-00004

Tanner, M. A., Travis, F., Gaylord-King, C., Haaga, D. A. F., Grosswald, S., & Schneider, R. H. (2009). The Effects of the Transcendental Meditation program on mindfulness. *Journal of Clinical Psychology, 65*(6), 574–589. https://doi.org/10.1002/jclp.20544

Targ, E. F., & Levine, E. G. (2002). The efficacy of a mind-body-spirit group for women with breast cancer: A randomized controlled trial. *General Hospital Psychiatry, 24*(4), 238–248. https://doi.org/10.1016/S0163-8343(02)00191-3

Teasdale, J. D., Segal, Z. V., Williams, J. M. G., Ridgeway, V. A., Soulsby, J. M., & Lau, M. A. (2000). Prevention of relapse/recurrence of major depression by Mindfulness-Based Cognitive Therapy. *Journal of Consulting and Clinical Psychology, 68*(4), 615–623. https://doi.org/10.1037/0022-006X.68.4.615

The Epoch Times. (2004). On the collusion of Jiang Zemin and the communist party to persecute Falun Gong. In *Nine Commentaries on the Communist Party* (pp. 115–147). Yih Chyun Corp.

The journey of Falun Dafa. (2002, July 2002). A photo exhibit of ten years since the introduction of Falun Dafa to the public. *Compassion Magazine*, 40–49.

Thompson, B. (2009). Personal communication with Adelaide Falun Dafa assistant: Ethnic diversity of the Falun Gong community in South Australia.

Thorndike, E. L. (1920). A constant error in psychological ratings. *Journal of Abnormal and Social Psychology, 41*(1), 258–290.

Tooley, G. A., Armstrong, S. M., Norman, T. R., & Sali, A. (2000). Acute increases in night-time plasma melatonin levels following a period of meditation. *Biological Psychology, 53*(1), 69–78. https://doi.org/10.1016/S0301-0511(00)00035-1

Tourangeau, R., Couper, M. P., & Steiger, D. M. (2003). Humanizing self-administered surveys: Experiments on social presence in web and IVR surveys. *Computers in Human Behavior, 19*(1), 1–24. https://doi.org/10.1016/S0747-5632(02)00032-8

Travis, J. W., & Ryan, R. S. (1988). *Wellness workbook* (2nd ed.). Ten Speed Press.

Tsang, H. W. H., Mok, C. K., Au-Yeung, Y. T., & Chan, S. Y. C. (2003). The effect of qigong on general and psychosocial health of elderly with chronic physical illness: A randomized clinical trial. *International Journal of Geriatic Psychiatry, 18*(5), 441–449. https://doi.org/10.1002/gps.861

Upchurch, D. M., Chyu, L., Greendale, G. A., Utts, J., Bair, Y. A., Zhang, G., et al. (2007). Complementary and alternative medicine use among American women: Findings from the National Health Interview Survey, 2002. *Journal of Women's Health, 16*(1), 102–113. https://doi.org/10.1089/jwh.2006.M074

Vadiraja, H. S., Rao, M. R., Nagarathna, R., Nagendra, H. R., Rekha, M., Vanitha, N., et al. (2009). Effects of yoga program on quality of life and affect in early breast cancer patients undergoing adjuvant radiotherapy: A randomized controlled trial. *Complementary Therapies in Medicine, 17*(5–6), 274–280. https://doi.org/10.1016/j.ctim.2009.06.004

VandenBos, G. R. (Ed.) (2007) *APA dictionary of psychology* (1st ed.). American Psychological Association.

Voukelatos, A., Cumming, R. G., Lord, S. R., & Rissel, C. (2007). A randomized, controlled trial of Tai Chi for the prevention of falls: The Central Sydney Tai Chi trial. *Journal of the American Geriatrics Society, 55*(8), 1185–1191. https://doi.org/10.1111/j.1532-5415.2007.01244.x

Wallis, C. (2005, January 17). The new science of happiness. *Time Magazine,* 43–49.

Walsh, R. (1989). Asian psychotherapies. In R. J. Corsini & D. Wedding (Eds.), *Current Psychotherapies* (4th ed., pp. 547–559). F. E. Peacock Publishers, Inc.

Walsh, R., & Bugental, J. (2005). Long-term benefits from psychotherapy: A 30-year retrospective by client and therapist. *Journal of Humanistic Psychology, 45*(4), 531–542. https://doi.org/10.1177/0022167805280266

Walsh, R., & Vaughan, F. (Eds.). (1993). *Paths beyond ego: The transpersonal vision.* Jeremy P. Tarcher/Perigee.

Wang, Q., Li, N., Zheng, L., Qu, e., Tian, X., & Jing, L. (1998). The effect of Falun Gong on healing illnesses and keeping fit: A sampling survey of practitioners from Beijing Zizhuyuan Assistance Center. http://en.minghui.org/eng/science_eng/survey98_2eng.htm

Ware Jr., J. E. (2000). SF-36 Health Survey update. *Spine, 25*(24), 3130–3139.

Ware Jr., J. E. (2008). SF-36® Health Survey update. Retrieved March 31, 2020, from https://www.researchgate.net/publication/12203625_SF-36_Health_Survey_update

Ware Jr., J. E., & Sherbourne, C. D. (1992). The MOS 36-Item Short-Form Health Survey (SF-36): I. Conceptual framework and item selection. *Medical Care, 30*(6), 473–483.

Weaver, A. J., Flannelly, L. T., Garbarino, J., Figley, C. R., & Flannelly, K. J. (2003). A systematic review of research on religion and spirituality in the *Journal of Traumatic Stress:* 1990–1999. *Mental Health, Religion & Culture, 6*(3), 215–228. https://doi.org/10.1080/1367467031000088123

Wessinger, C. (2003). Falun Gong symposium introduction and glossary. *Nova Religio: The Journal of Alternative and Emergent Religions, 6*(2), 215–222. https://doi.org/10.1525/nr.2003.6.2.215

Westphal, T. (1989). Wellness models. In P. A. Swinford & J. A. Webster (Eds.), *Promoting Wellness: A nurse's handbook* (pp. 302). Aspen Publishers, Inc.

What is Falun Dafa? (2002, July 2002). What is Falun Dafa? An introduction. *Compassion Magazine*, 70–71.

Williams, D. R., & Sternthal, M. J. (2007). Spirituality, religion and health: Evidence and research directions. *The Medical Journal of Australia, 186*(10), S47–S50. https://doi.org/10.5694/j.1326-5377.2007.tb01040.x

Wilson, L. (2011). *Retracing, healing reactions and flare-ups.* Moses Nutrition. http://www.mosesnutrition.com/forms_and_articles/retracing-healing-reactions-or-flare-ups/

Winseman, A. L. (2002a). *Religion and gender: A congregation divided.* Gallup. http://www.gallup.com/poll/7336/Religion-Gender-Congregation-Divided.aspx

Winseman, A. L. (2002b). *Religion and gender: A congregation divided, Part II.* Gallup. http://www.gallup.com/poll/7390/Religion-Gender-Congregation-Divided-Part.aspx

Winseman, A. L. (2003). *Spiritual commitment by age and gender.* Gallup. http://www.gallup.com/poll/7963/Spiritual-Commitment-Age-Gender.aspx

Witmer, J. M., & Sweeney, T. J. (1992). A holistic model for wellness and prevention over the life span. *Journal of Counseling & Development, 71*(2), 140–148.

Wolsko, P. M., Eisenberg, D. M., Davis, R. B., Ettner, S. L., & Phillips, R. S. (2002). Insurance coverage, medical conditions, and visits to alternative medicine providers. *Archives of Internal Medicine, 162*(3), 281–287. https://doi.org/10.1001/archinte.162.3.281

Wolsko, P. M., Eisenberg, D. M., Davis, R. B., & Phillips, R. S. (2004). Use of mind-body medical therapies. *Journal of General Internal Medicine, 19*(1), 43–50. https://doi.org/10.1111/j.1525-1497.2004.21019.x

World Health Organization. (2003). *The World Health Organization: Definition of health. WHO.* Retrieved July 16, 2008, from https://8fit.com/lifestyle/the-world-health-organization-definition-of-health/

World Health Organization. (2007). *Mental health: Strengthening mental health promotion.* Retrieved July 16, 2008, from https://mindyourmindproject.org/wp-content/uploads/2014/11/WHO-Statement-on-Mental-Health-Promotion.pdf

World Organization to Investigate the Persecution of Falun Gong. (2004). *Investigation report on the persecution of Falun Gong: Volume 1* (2nd ed.). World Organization to Investigate the Persecution of Falun Gong (WOIPFG).

Wu, P., Fuller, C., Liu, X., Lee, H.-C., Fan, B., Hoven, C. W., et al. (2007). Use of complementary and alternative medicine among women with depression: Results of a national survey. *Psychiatric Services, 58*(3), 349–356. https://doi.org/10.1176/appi.ps.58.3.349

Xie, F. T., & Zhu, T. (2004). *Ancient wisdom for modern predicaments: The truth, deceit, and issues surrounding Falun Gong.* Presented at the American Family Foundation Conference, in Enfield, Connecticut, October 17-18, 2003. *Cultic Studies Review.* http://franktianxie.blog.epochtimes.com/article/show?articleid=4511

Xu, J. (1999). Body, discourse, and the cultural politics of contemporary Chinese Qigong. *The Journal of Asian Studies, 58*(4), 961–991. https://doi.org/10.2307/2658492

Yang, J. D. (2003). Falun Dafa—A science of body, mind and spirit. http://en.minghui.org/emh/download/publications/enlighten_2.html

Yang, J. D., & Nania, J. (2001). Falun Dafa: Health benefits, anti-aging, and beyond. https://www.pureinsight.org/node/154

Yeager, D. M., Glei, D. A., Au, M., Lin, H., Sloan, R. P., & Weinstein, M. (2006). Religious involvement and health outcomes among older persons in Taiwan. *Social Science & Medicine, 63*(8), 2228–2241. https://doi.org/10.1016/j.socscimed.2006.05.007

Yeh, G. Y., Davis, R. B., & Phillips, R. S. (2006). Use of complementary therapies in patients with cardiovascular disease. *The American Journal of Cardiology, 98*(5), 673–680. https://doi.org/10.1016/j.amjcard.2006.03.051

Yeh, G. Y., Wood, M. J., Lorell, B. H., Stevenson, L. W., Eisenberg, D. M., Wayne, P. M., et al. (2004). Effects of Tai Chi mind-body movement therapy on functional status and exercise capacity in patients with chronic heart failure: A randomized controlled trial. *The American Journal of Medicine, 117*(8), 541–548. https://doi.org/10.1016/j.amjmed.2004.04.016

Zeidan, F., Gordon, N. S., Merchant, J., & Goolkasian, P. (2009). The effects of brief mindfulness meditation training on experimentally induced pain. *The Journal of Pain, 11*(3) 199–209. https://doi.org/10.1016/j.jpain.2009.07.015

Zhang, R., & Xiao, J. (1996). A report on the effect of Falun Gong in curing diseases and keeping fit based on a survey of 355 cultivators of Falun Gong at certain sites in Beijing, China. Retrieved December 17, 2003, from www.falundafa-pa.net/survey/survey96_e.pdf

Zollman, C., & Vickers, A. (1999). What is complementary medicine? *British Medical Journal, 319*(7211), 693–696. https://doi.org/10.1136/bmj.319.7211.693

Zylowska, L., Ackerman, D. L., Yang, M. H., Futrell, J. L., Horton, N. L., Hale, T. S., et al. (2008). Mindfulness meditation training in adults and adolescents with ADHD: A feasibility study. *Journal of Attention Disorders, 11*(6), 737–746. https://doi.org/10.1177/1087054707308502

Updated Resources

Behrens, A. (2017). *Falun Gong in der Schule—Motive, Umsetzungsformen, und Erfahrungen* (Falun Gong in schools—motives, implementation forms, and experiences). Master's thesis. University of Hildesheim, Germany. https://www.researchgate.net/publication/318300324_Falun_Gong_in_der_Schule_-_Motive_Umsetzungsformen_und_Erfahrungen

Bendig, B. W. (2013). *Cognitive and physiological effects of Falun Gong qigong.* [Doctoral dissertation, University of California, Los Angeles]. ProQuest ID: Bendig_ucla_0031D_11049. https://escholarship.org/uc/item/4899m047

Bendig, B. W., Shapiro, D., & Zaidel, E. (2020). Group differences between practitioners and novices in hemispheric processing of attention and emotion before and after a session of Falun Gong qigong. *Brain and Cognition, 138*, 105494. https://doi.org/10.1016/j.bandc.2019.105494

Cheung, M., Trey, T., Matas, D., & An, R. (2018). Cold Genocide: Falun Gong in China. *Genocide Studies and Prevention: An International Journal, 12*(1), 38–62. https://doi.org/10.5038/1911-9933.12.1.1513

Gutmann, E. (2014). *The slaughter: Mass killings, organ harvesting, and China's secret solution to its dissident problem.* Prometheus Books.

Trey, M. (2016). The study of the health-wellness effects of Falun Gong: Applications to counseling. *Spirituality and counseling issues: Vistas 2016, Article 25.* http://www.counseling.org/docs/default-source/vistas/articl e_2558c224f16116603abcacff0000bee5e7.pdf?sfvrsn=6

Trey, M. (2017). Falun Gong and its applications to counseling: Case examples. *Vistas 2017, Article 51.* https://www.counseling.org/docs/default-source/vistas/falun_gong.pdf?sfvrsn=4

Trey, M. (2017). *With wings, will fly: A spiritually integrated approach with Falun Gong.* Paper presented at the 2nd International Conference on Spirituality and Psychology, March 13–15, 2017. Bangkok, Thailand.

Trey, M. (2017). Hearts Uplifted Project: Documenting lived experiences of Falun Gong practitioners to examine their health, wellness, and resilience. (Unpublished research).

Trey, M. (2017). *Changing perceptions: An integrated approach with Falun Gong.* Presented at The International Conference on Social and Behavioral Sciences, August 14-16, 2017. Singapore.

Trey, M. (2018). Changing perceptions: An integrative approach with Falun Gong. *Advance Science Letters. 24*(5) pp.3469-3474. https://doi.org/10.1166/asl.2018.11414

Trey, M. (2018). *Therapy sans therapists: Overcoming anxiety, depression, and post-traumatic stress disorder with Falun Gong.* Invited to present at the 3rd International Conference on Spirituality and Psychology, March 13-15, 2018. Bangkok, Thailand.

Trey, M. (in press). *The mindful practice of Falun Gong: Meditation for health, wellness and beyond* (2nd ed.). First ed., 2016. Sibubooks LLC.

Trey, M. (2020). The Mindful Way of Falun Gong for graceful and positive aging. *Journal of Religion, Spirituality & Aging,* 1-16. Retrieved December 3, 2020 from https://doi.org/10.1080/15528030.2020.1847238

Trey, M., & Milner, C. (2017). A preliminary study exploring the extent Falun Gong practitioners who are health professionals integrate the practice with their work. [Unpublished raw data].

Trey, M., & Olatunji, C. (2019). *Use of Falun Gong to address traumatic stress among marginalized clients.* Invited to present at the 4th International Conference on Spirituality and Psychology, March 13–15, 2019. Bangkok, Thailand.

Trey, M., & Olatunji, C. (2020). Use of Falun Gong to address traumatic stress among marginalized clients. In Lobera, I. J. (Ed.), *Psychosomatic Medicine.* IntechOpen. https://doi.org/10.5772/intechopen.93301

Trey, M. & Zhang, D.X. (2020). *Using Falun Gong for achieving peace and conflict resolution.* Invited to present at the 7th Peace and Conflict Resolution virtual Conference, Dec 3–5, 2020. https://youtu.be/QNgBtcwwdY8

Won, X. (2017, October 25). Integrating Falun Gong into Western Counselling and Therapy. *The Epoch Times.*

Wu, S., Jiang, L., & Wang, J. (2017). From Relaxation Response, building power for health to an advanced self-cultivation practice: Genuine well-being. In Mollaoglu, M. (Ed.), *Well-being and Quality of Life—Medical Perspective.* IntechOpen. https://doi.org/10.5772/intechopen.68678

Index

About the Author

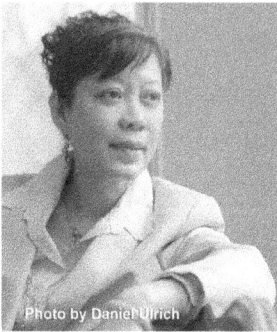

Photo by Daniel Ulrich

Sarawak-born Australian Dr. Margaret Trey lives in scenic Mid-Hudson region north of New York City with her Italian-speaking German-born husband. Inspired by her late author granduncle, she majored in English at The University of Toronto and completed the Doctorate of Counseling at The University of South Australia. Dr. Trey's upbringing profoundly impacted her affinity for traditional culture. Her maternal grandfather was a 19th century-born Taoist cultivator, healer, and physician. From her mother, who passed away at 103 years old, Dr. Trey learned the spirit and wisdom of traditional Chinese culture. An inherent respect for antiquated wisdom inspired Dr. Trey to study oriental medicine, Zen shiatsu, Indian and Japanese yoga, the yin-yang of foods, and Vipassana meditation—before she began practicing Falun Gong in 1997. Family lineage and belief in mind-body-spiritual approach have enthused Dr. Trey's integrated approach towards helping others. She creates ripples—of hope and positivity—through speaking at various events and international conferences in Australia, Canada, Singapore, Thailand, and the United States, as well as through her writings. Counselor, researcher, speaker, and author of two books on the effects of Falun Gong, Dr. Trey is currently focusing on her third book, *The Link between Falun Gong and Health–The Belief Factor* and collecting data for the fourth book.

Follow her on Facebook, Twitter @DrMTrey, and visit her author website www.margarettrey.com for anecdotes, reflections on nurturing a mindful, healthful lifestyle, and news about forthcoming books.

.